# THE PICTURE BOOK OF

# DOGS

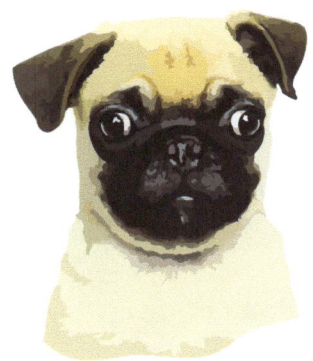

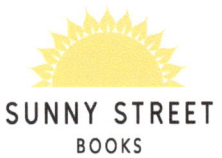

SUNNY STREET

BOOKS

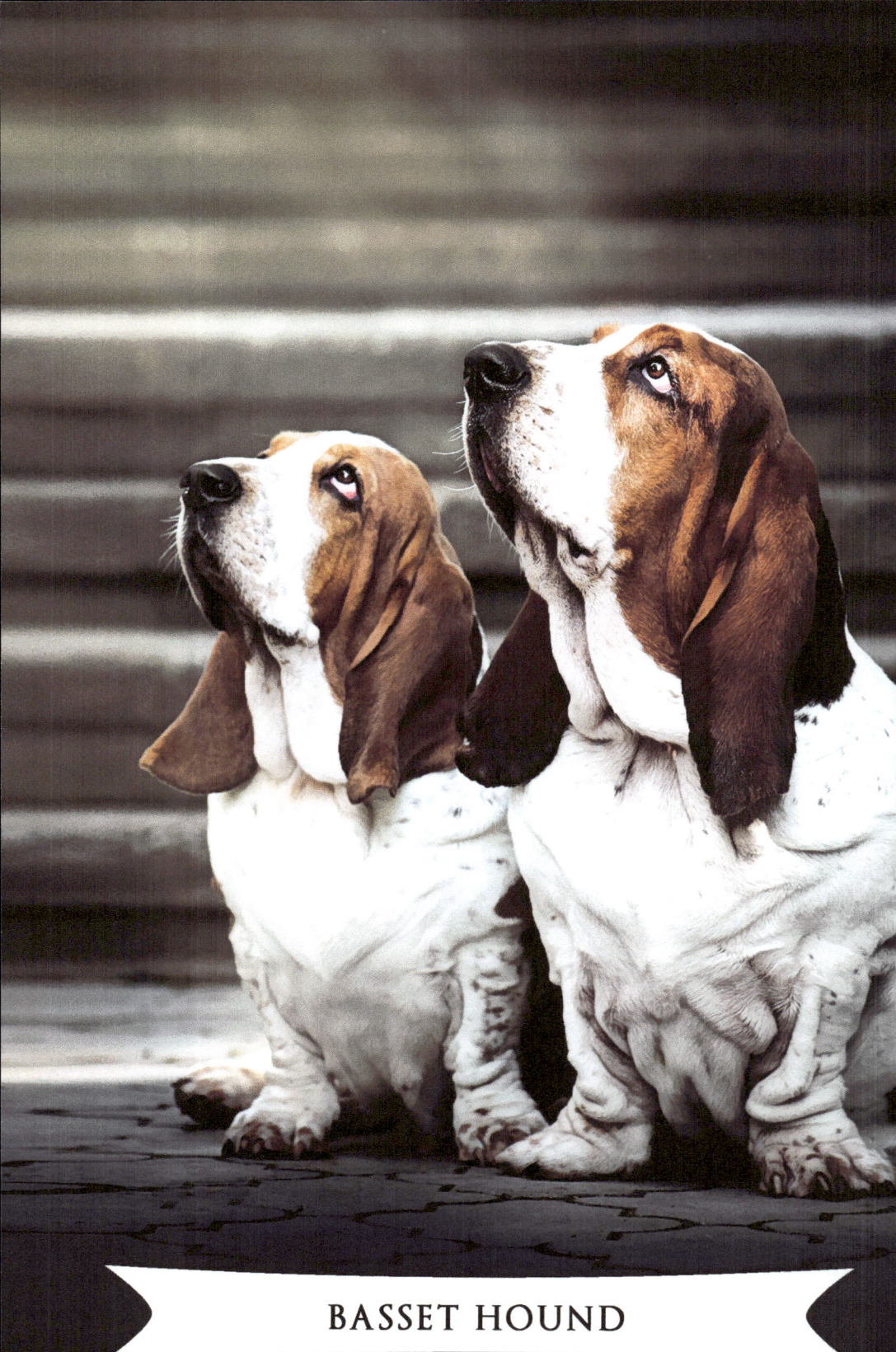

BASSET HOUND

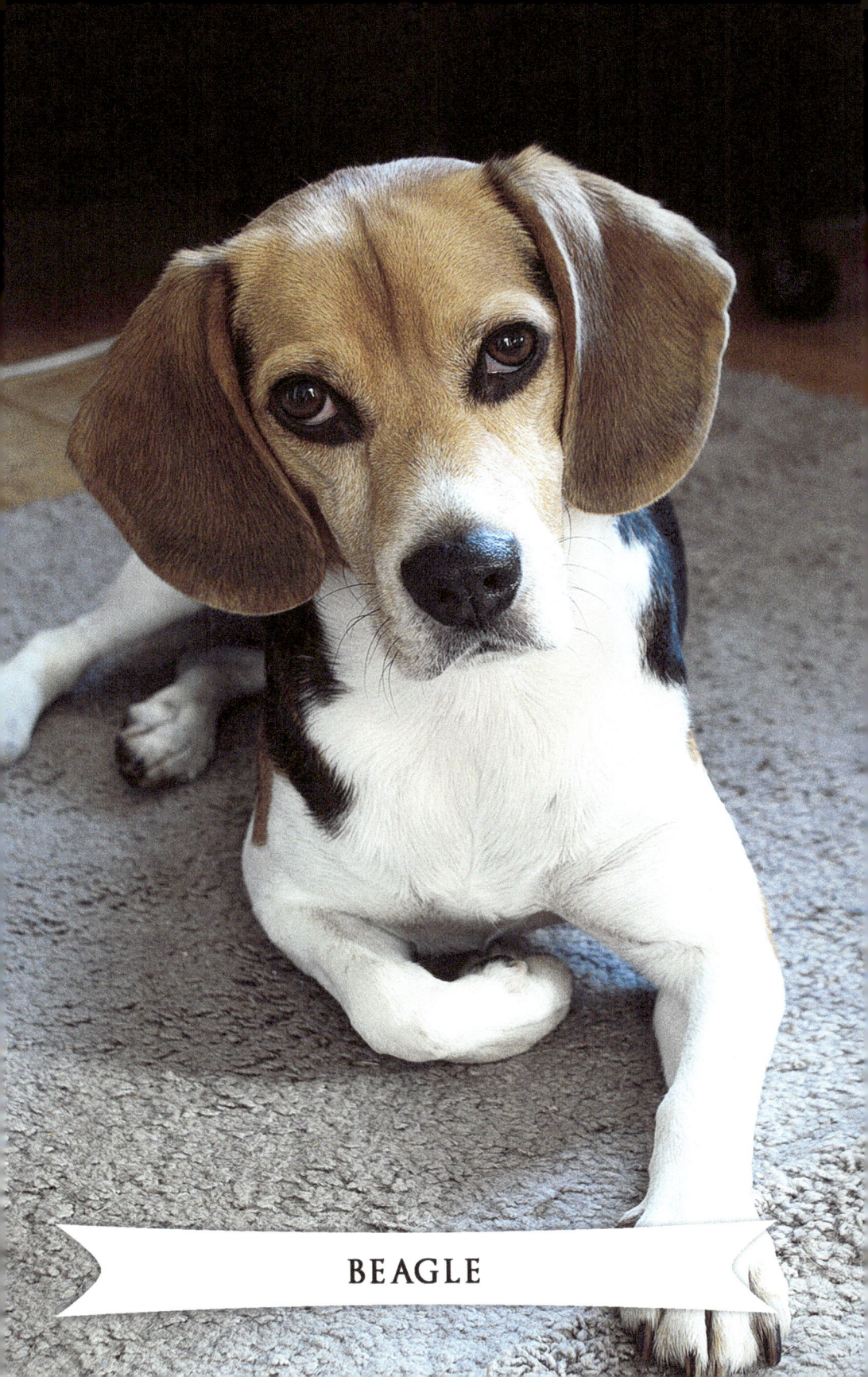

BEAGLE

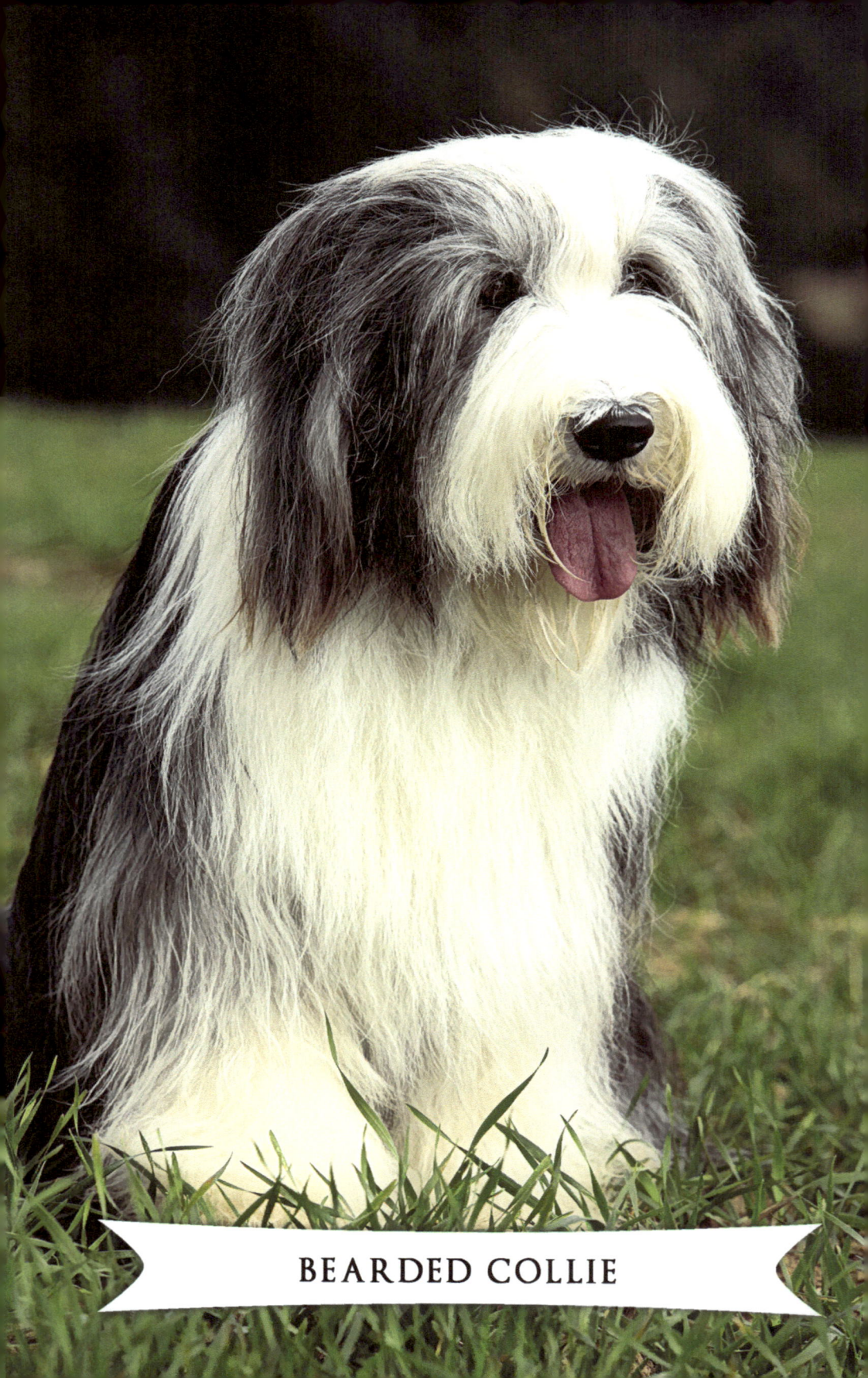

BEARDED COLLIE

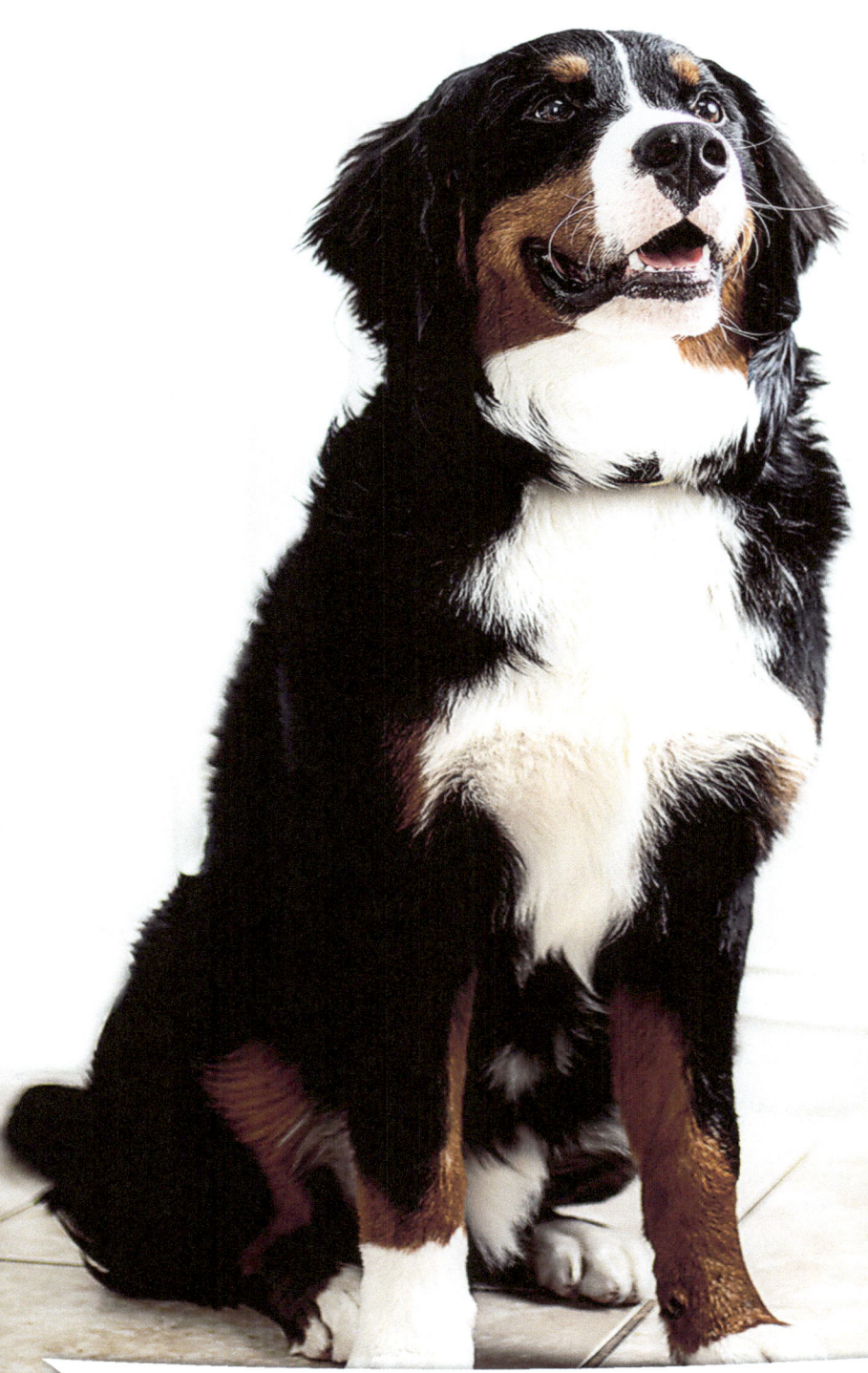

BERNESE MOUNTAIN DOG

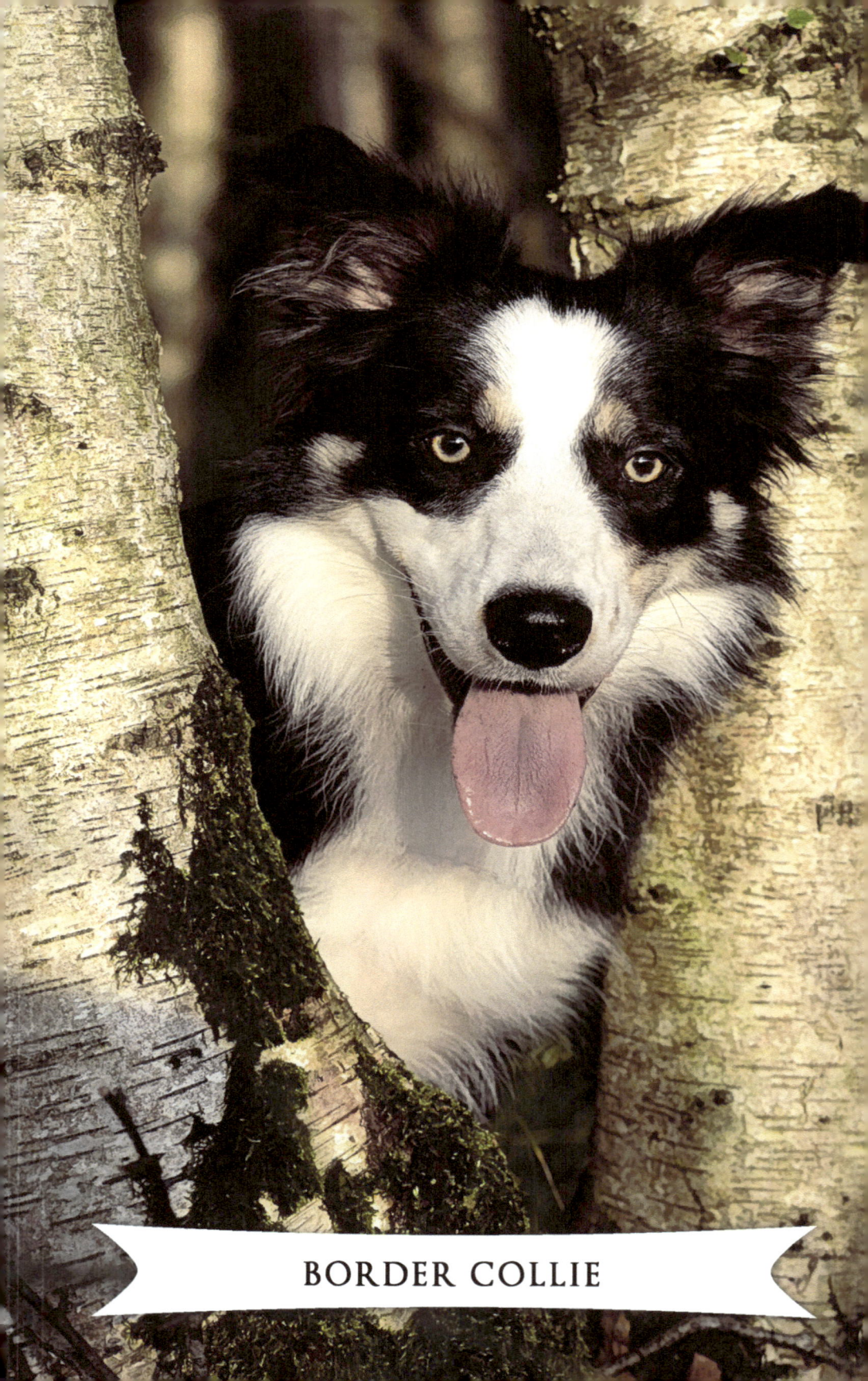

BORDER COLLIE

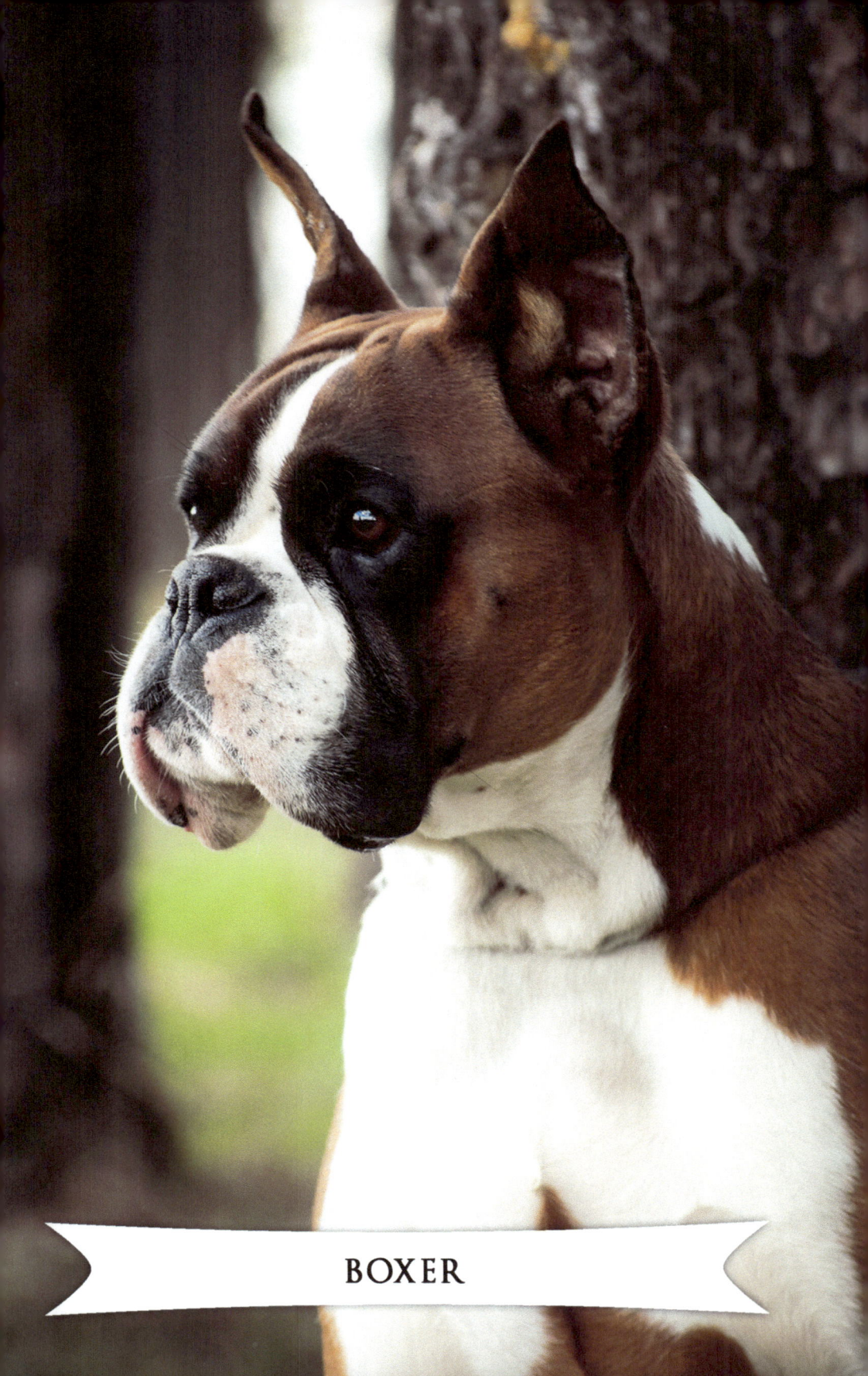

BOXER

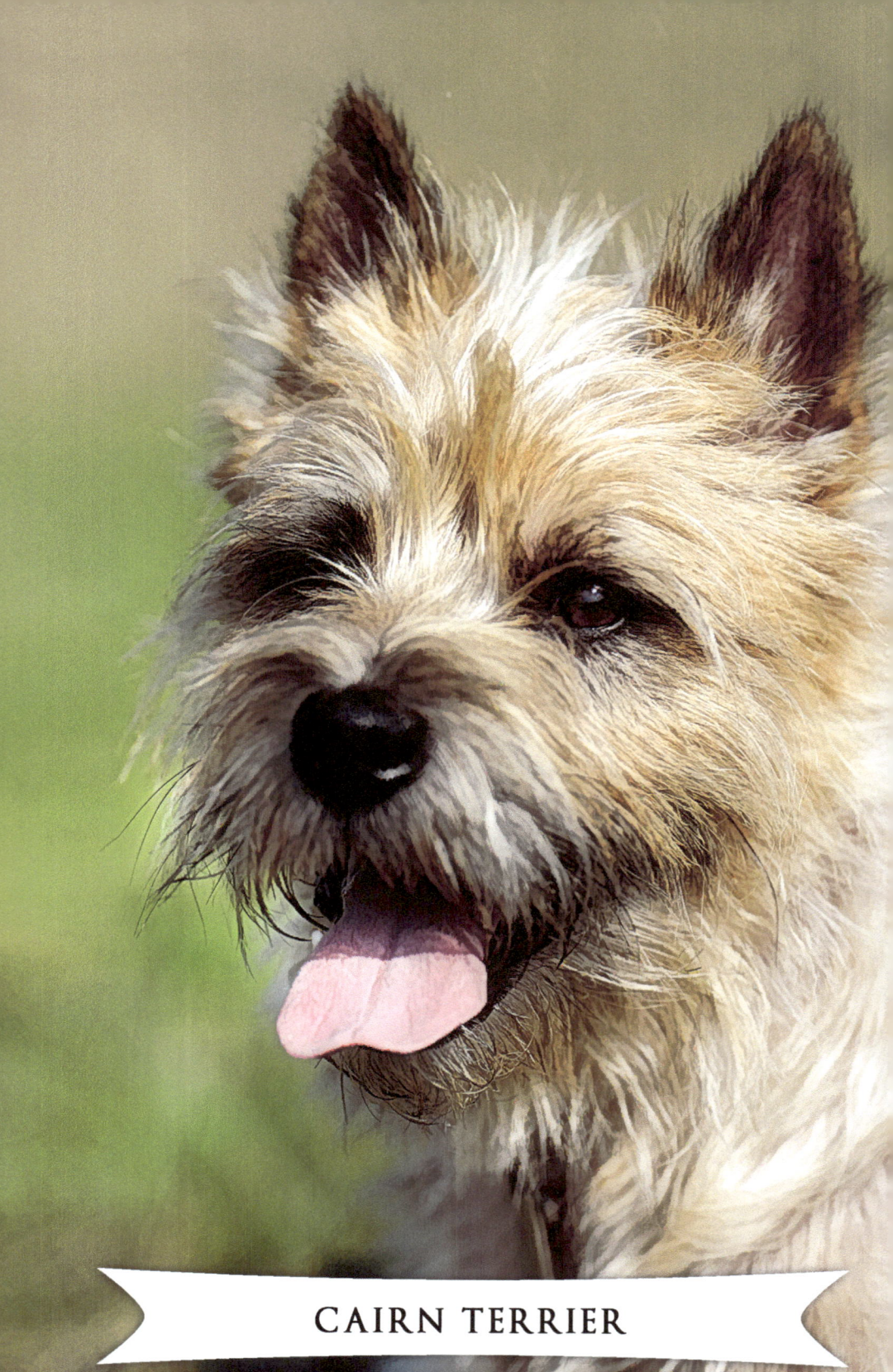

CAIRN TERRIER

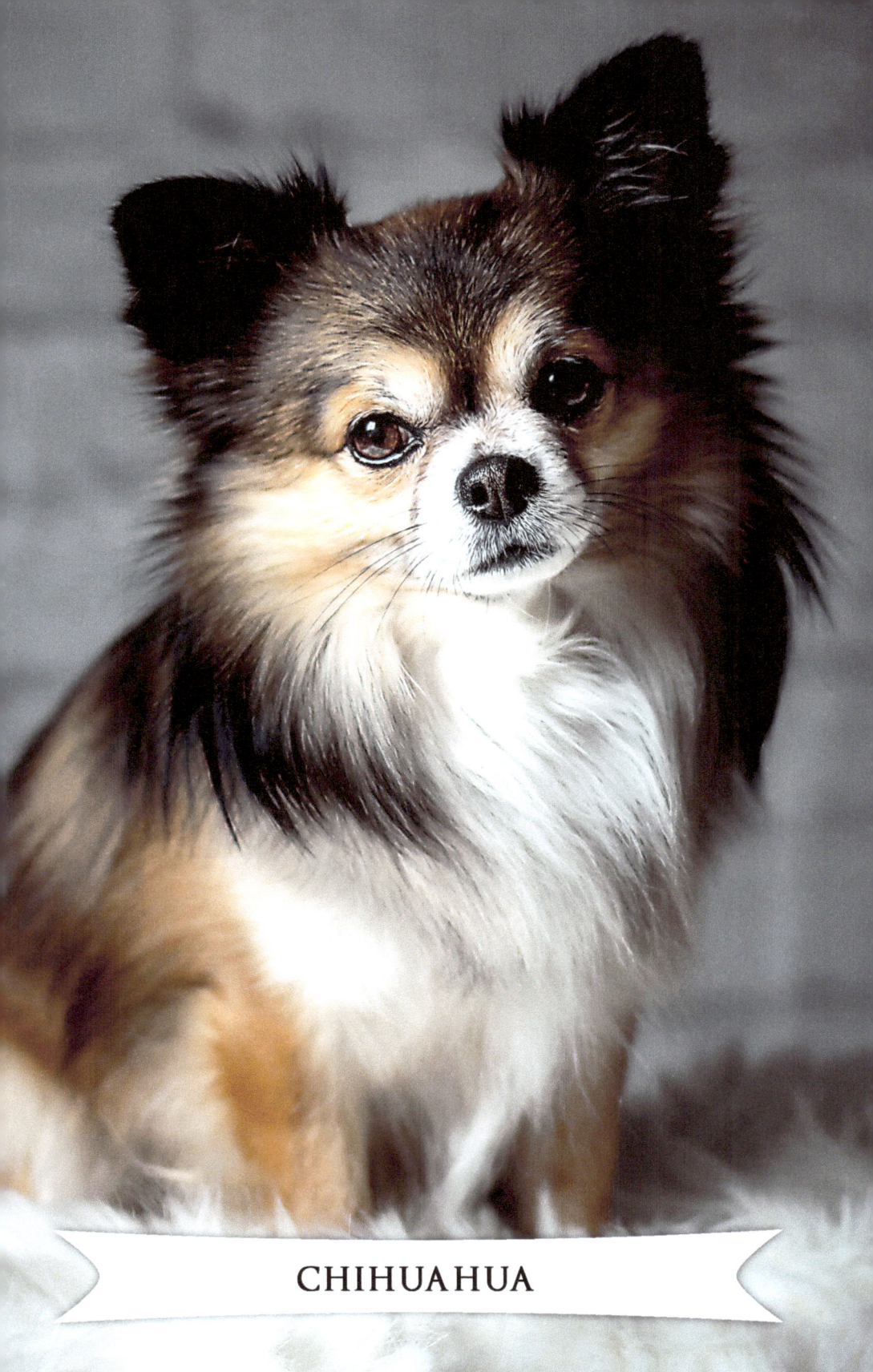

CHIHUAHUA

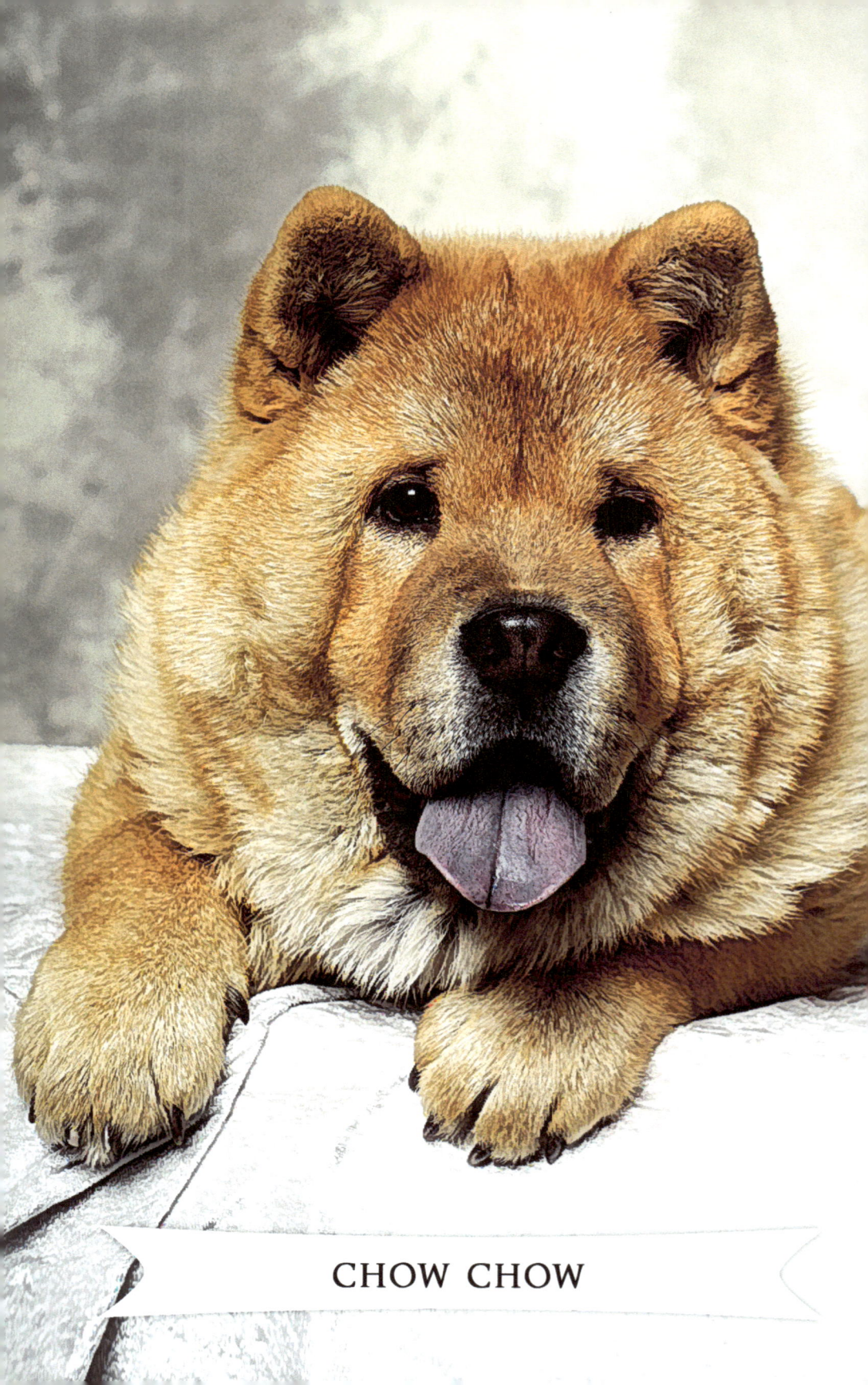

CHOW CHOW

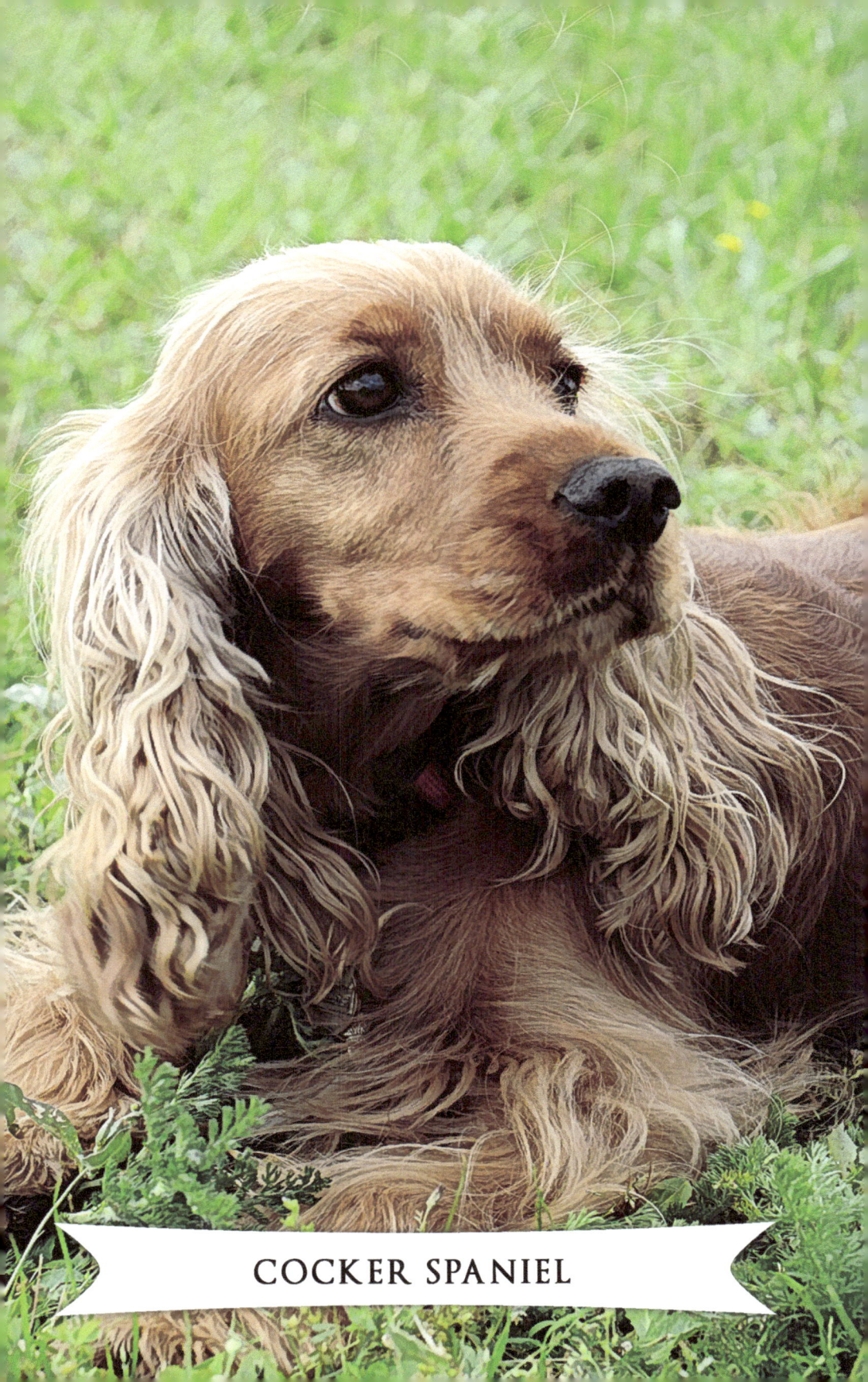

COCKER SPANIEL

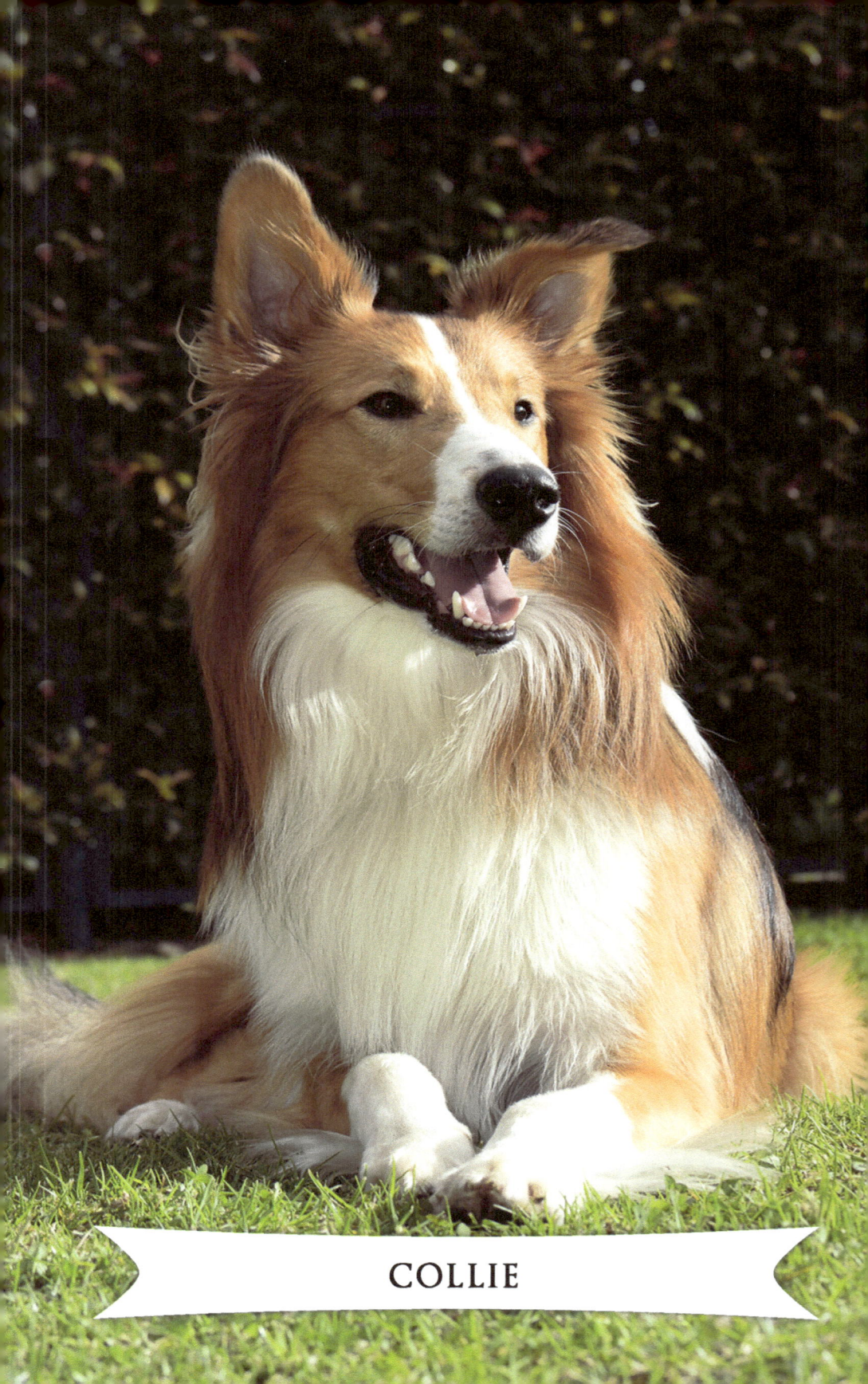

COLLIE

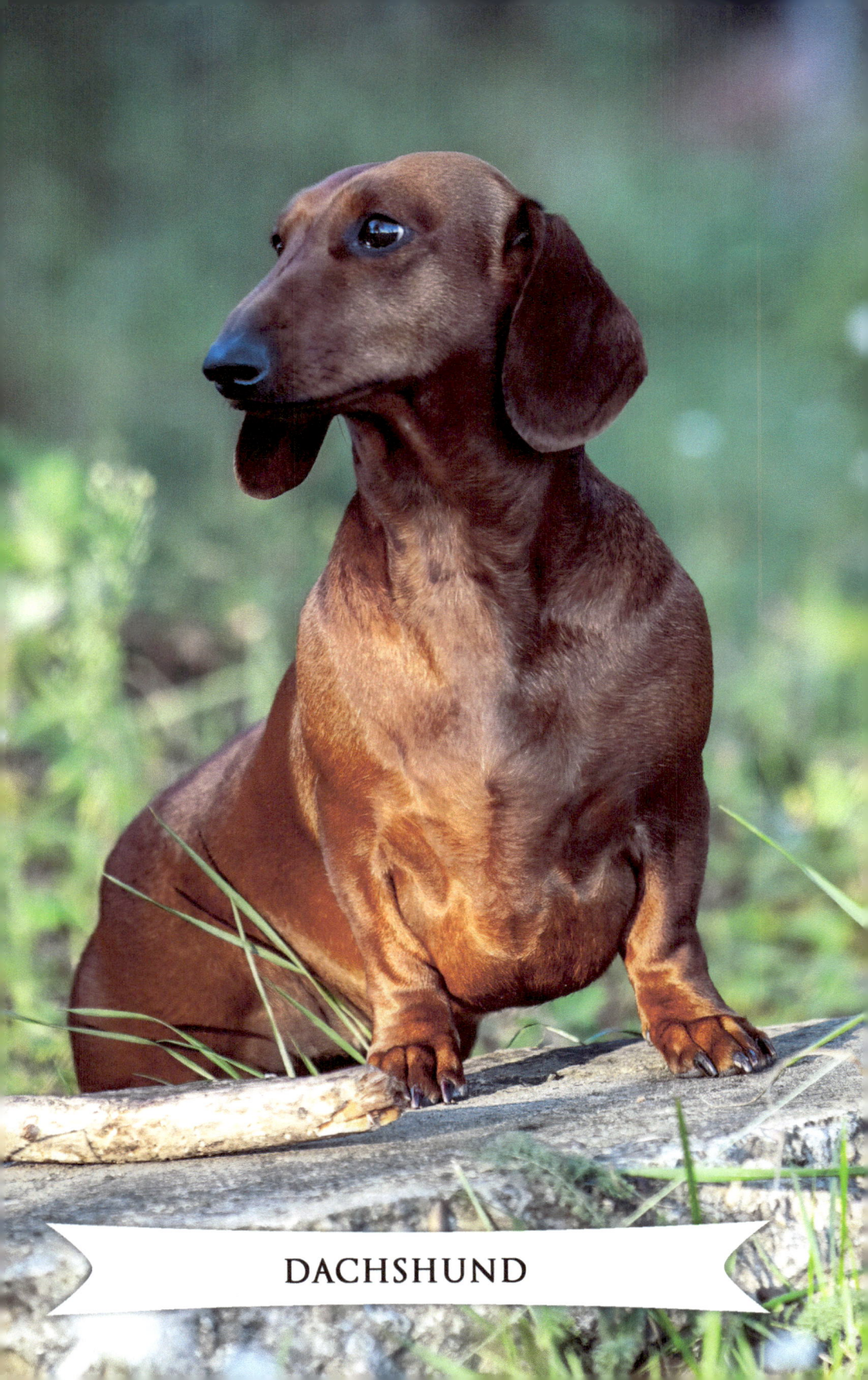

DACHSHUND

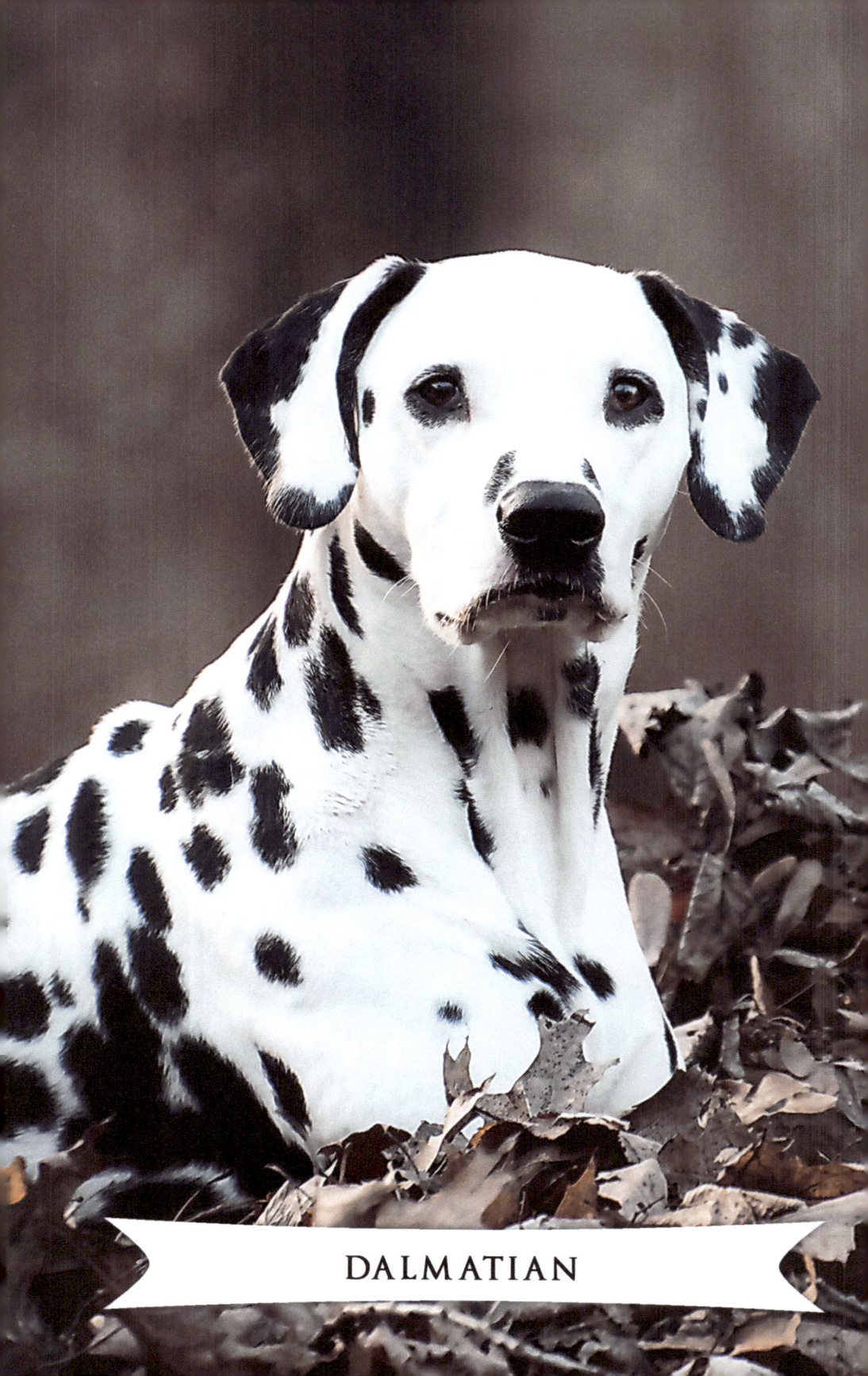

DALMATIAN

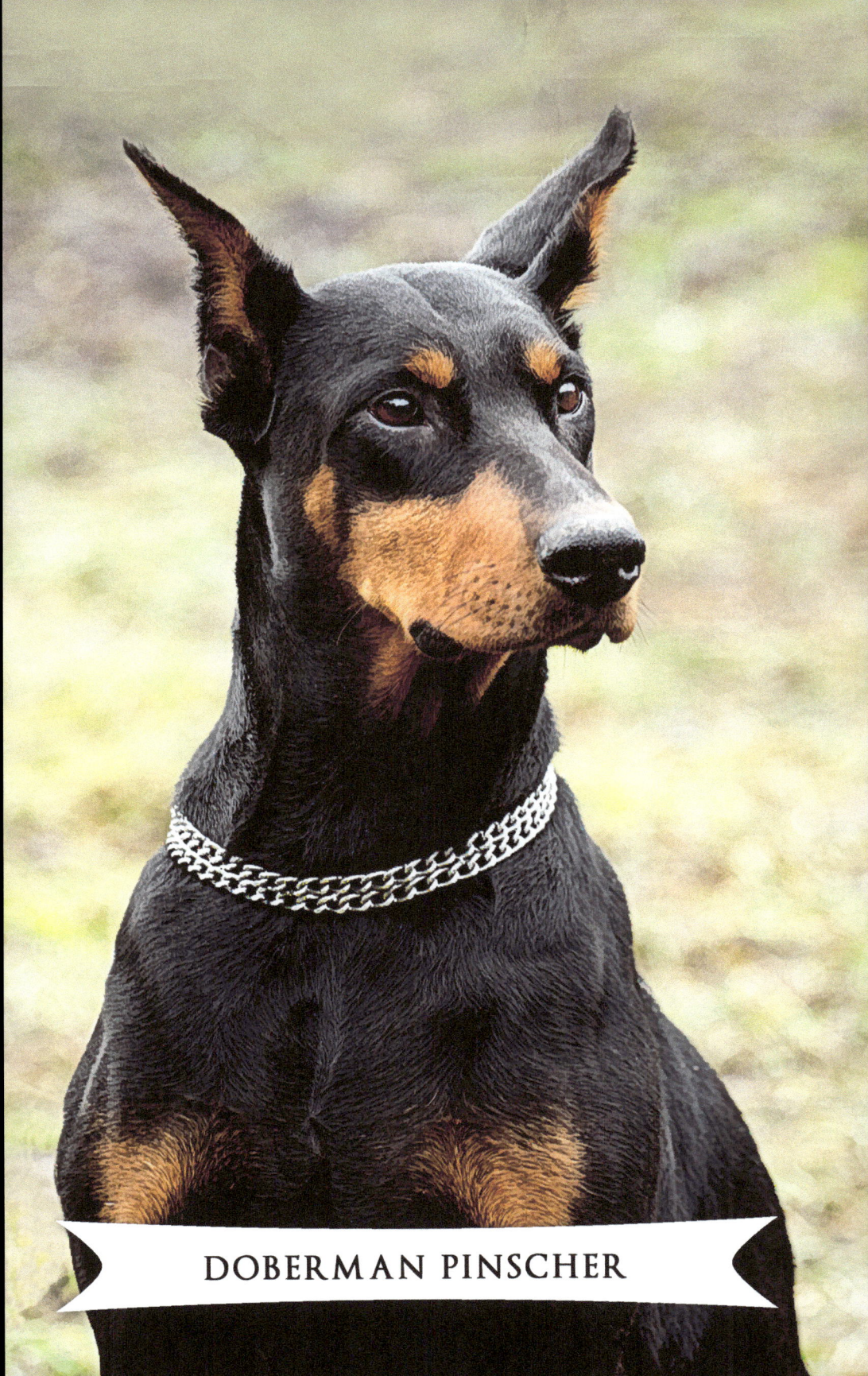

DOBERMAN PINSCHER

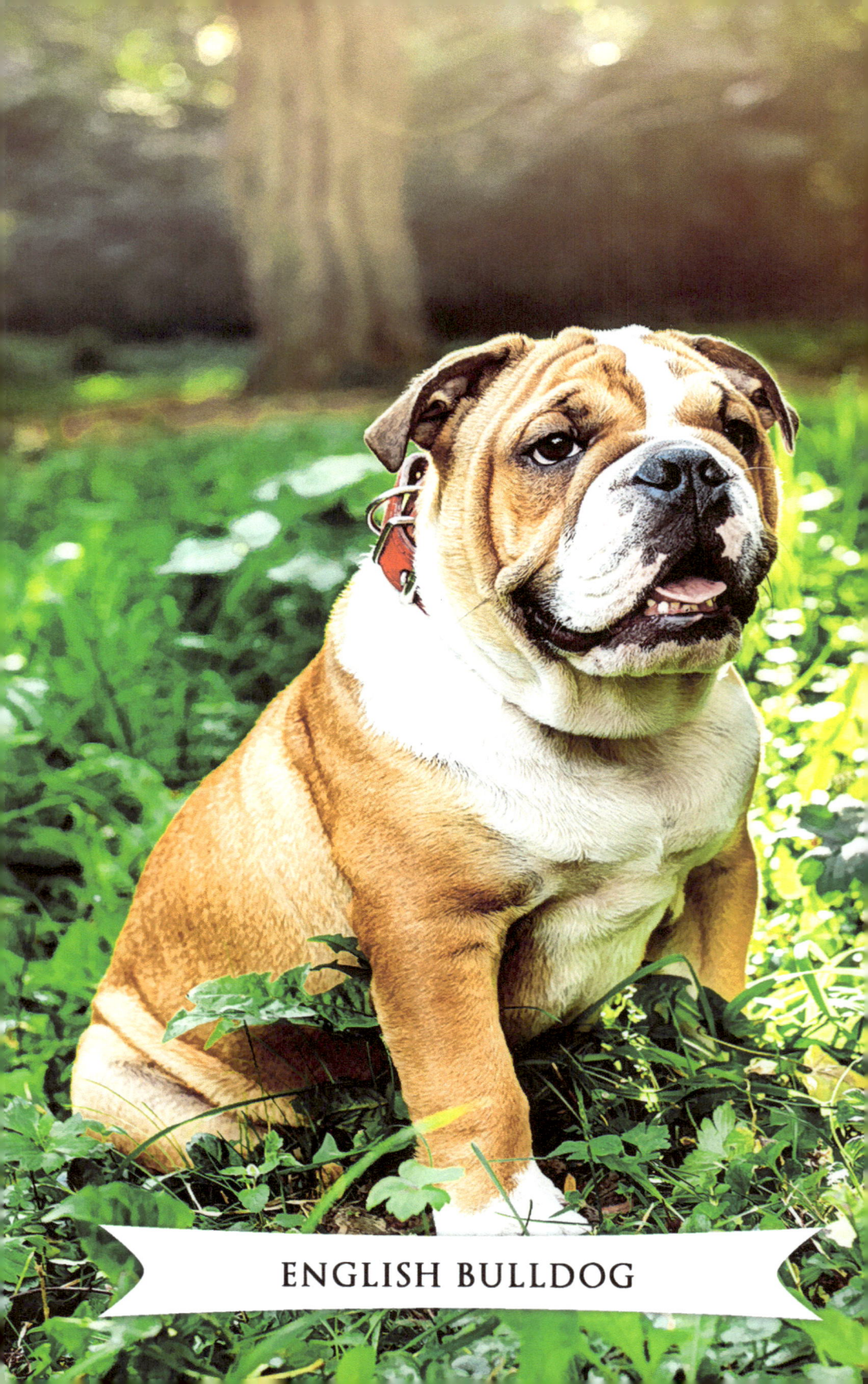

ENGLISH BULLDOG

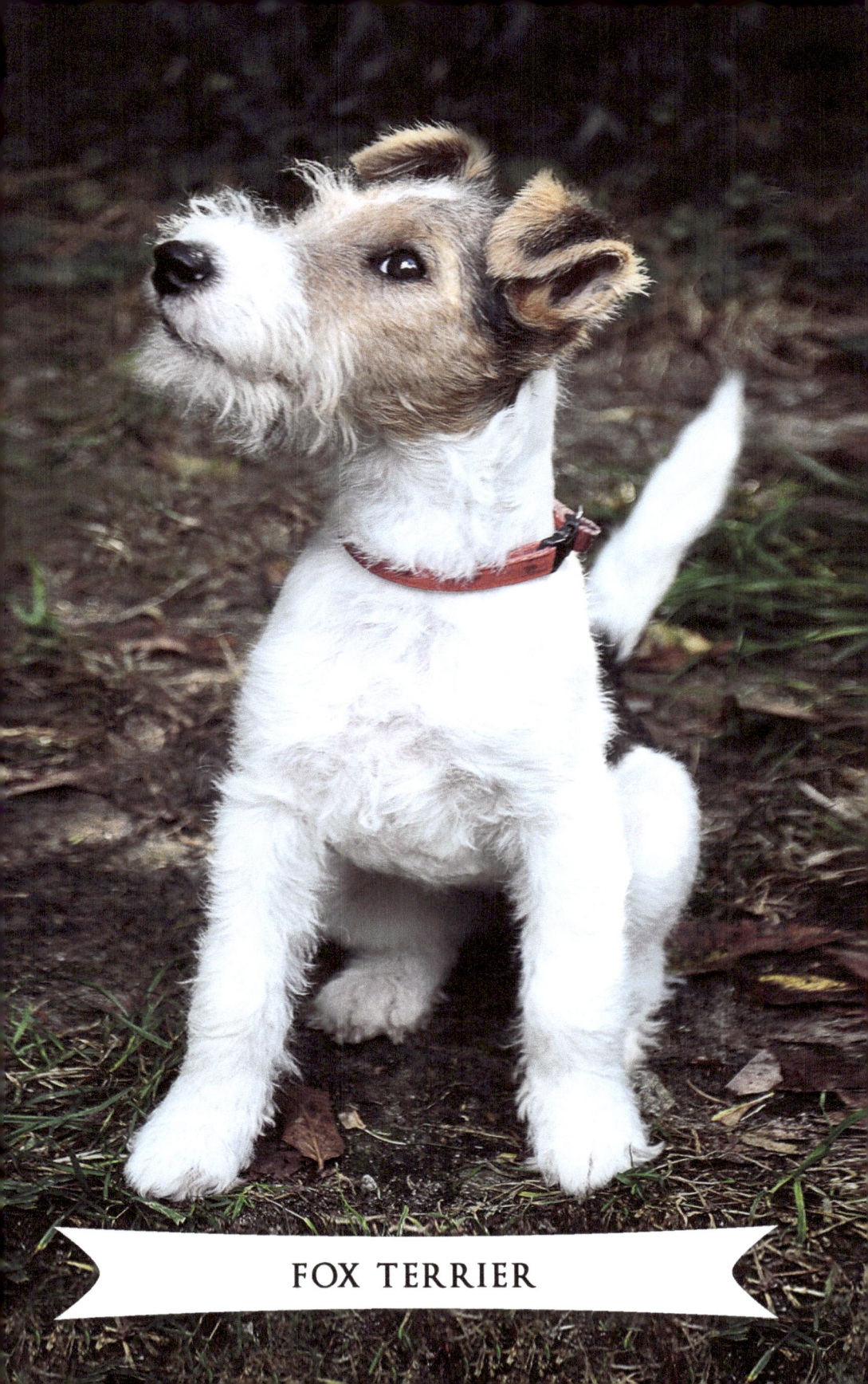

FOX TERRIER

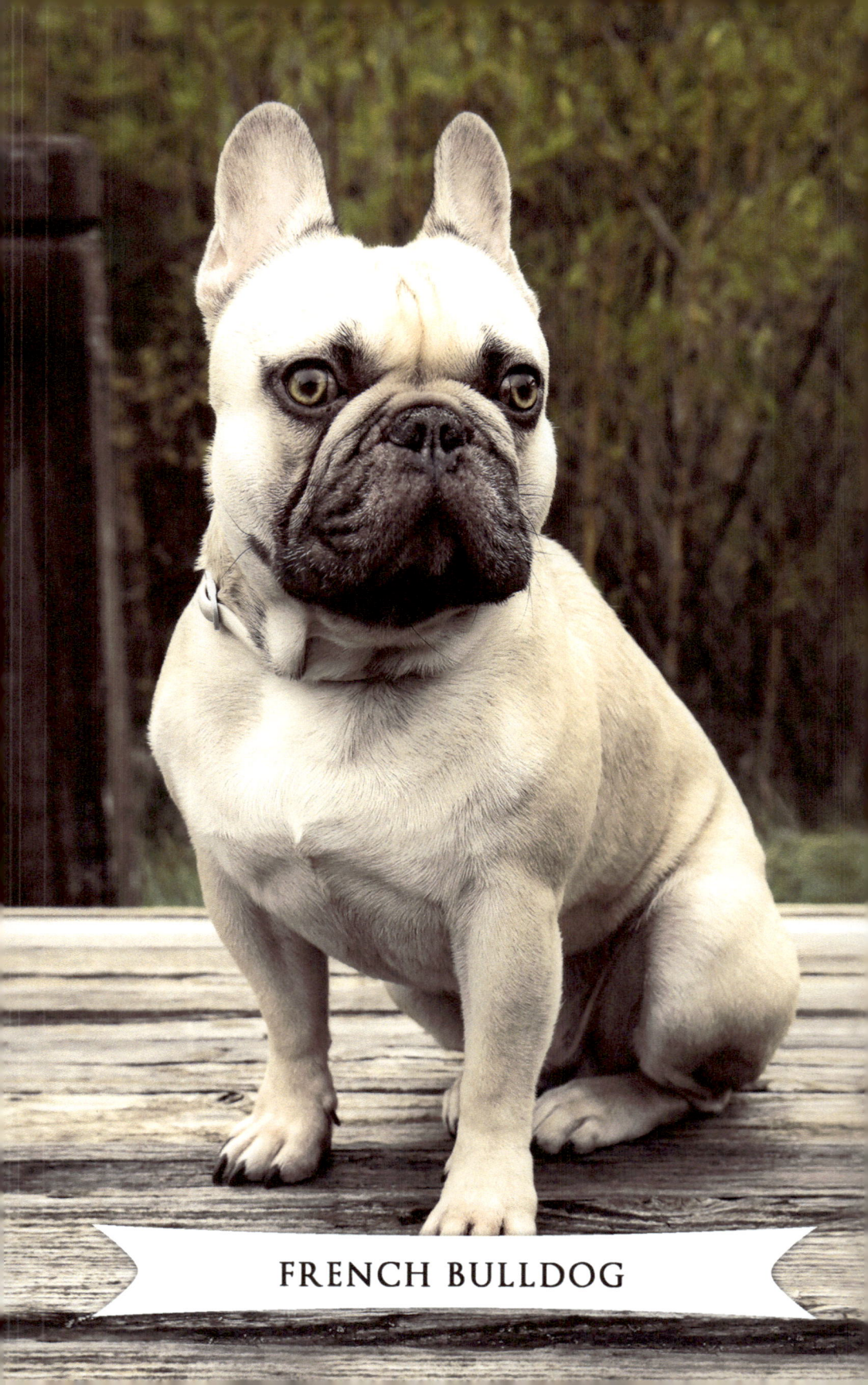

FRENCH BULLDOG

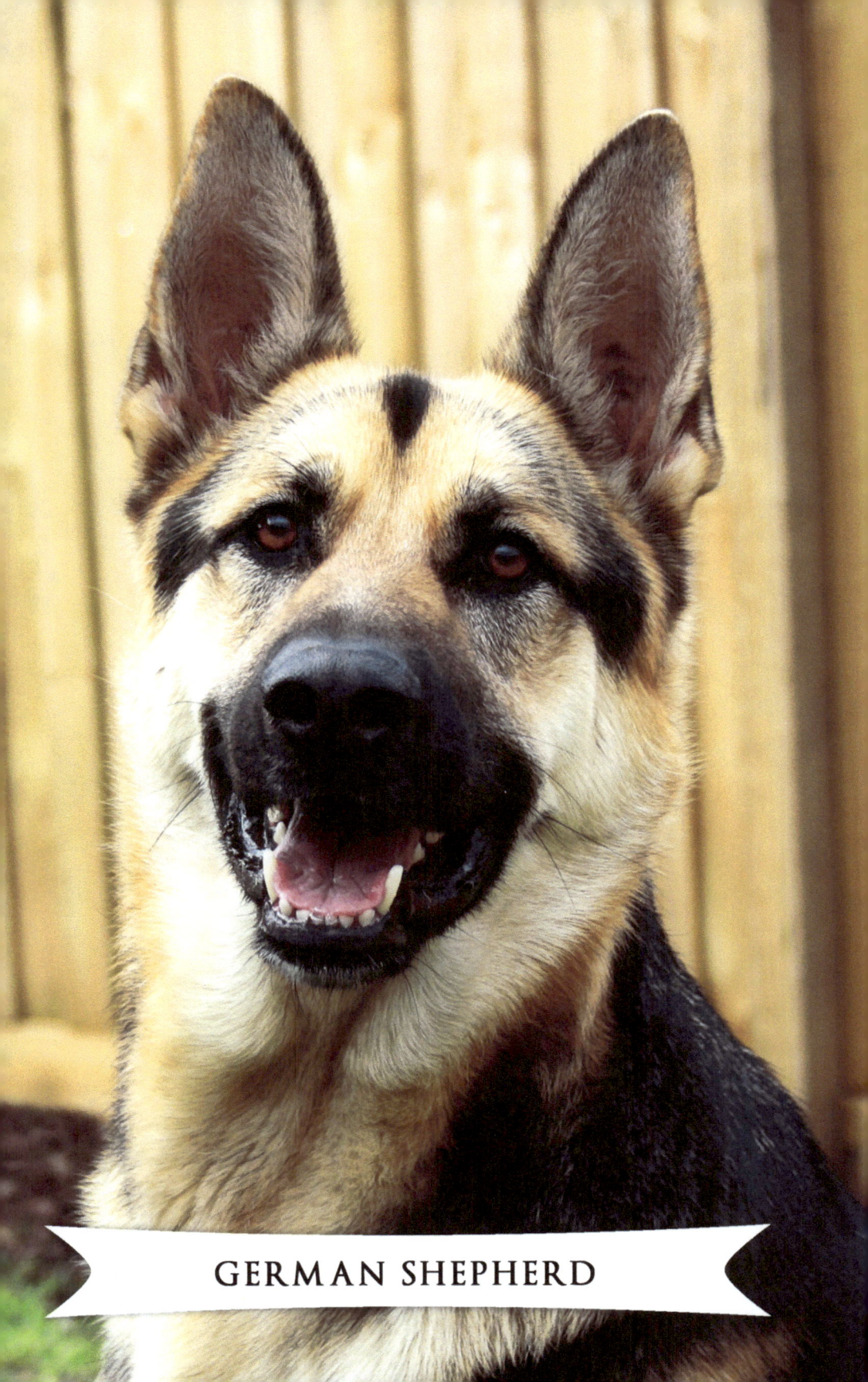

GERMAN SHEPHERD

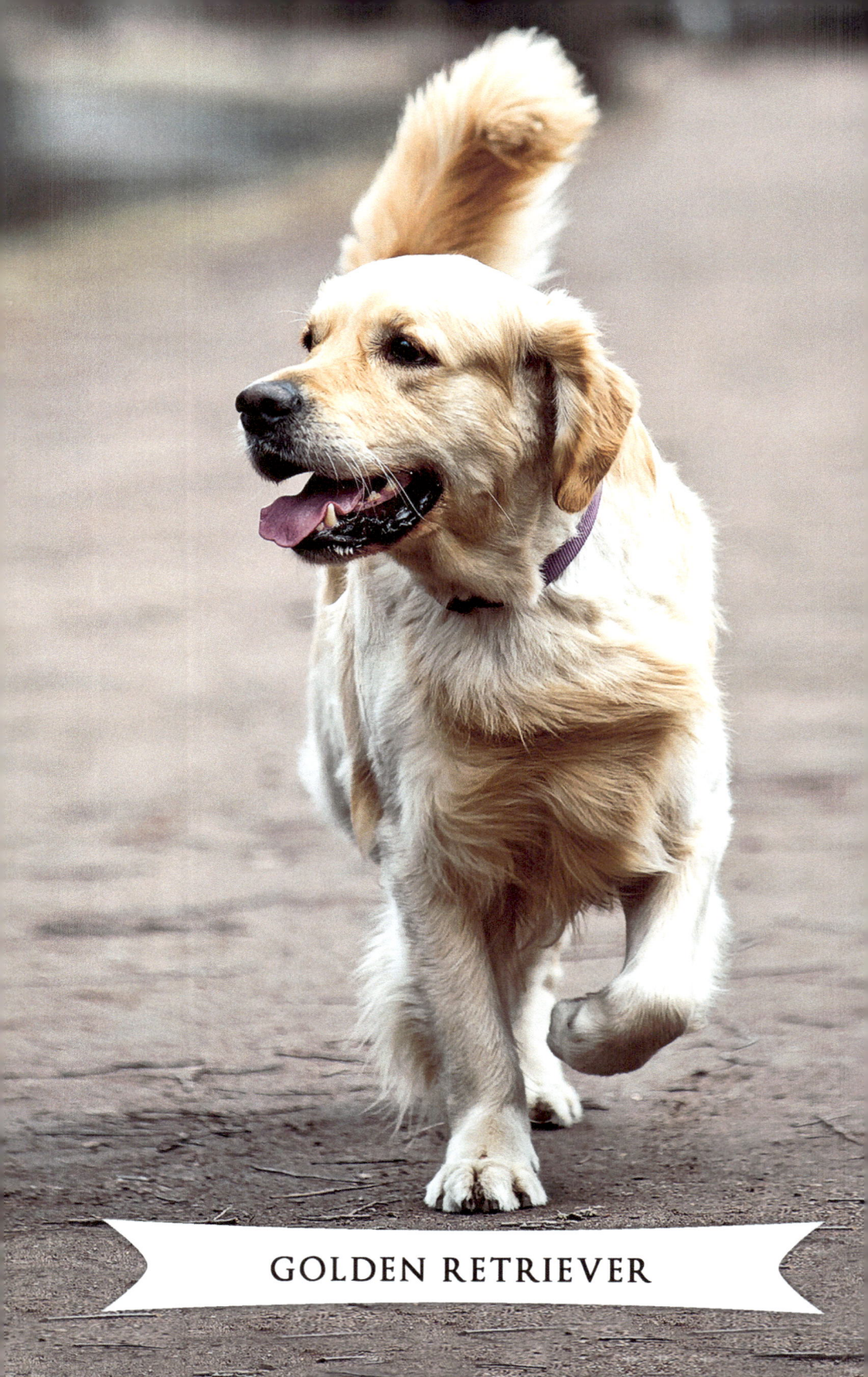

GOLDEN RETRIEVER

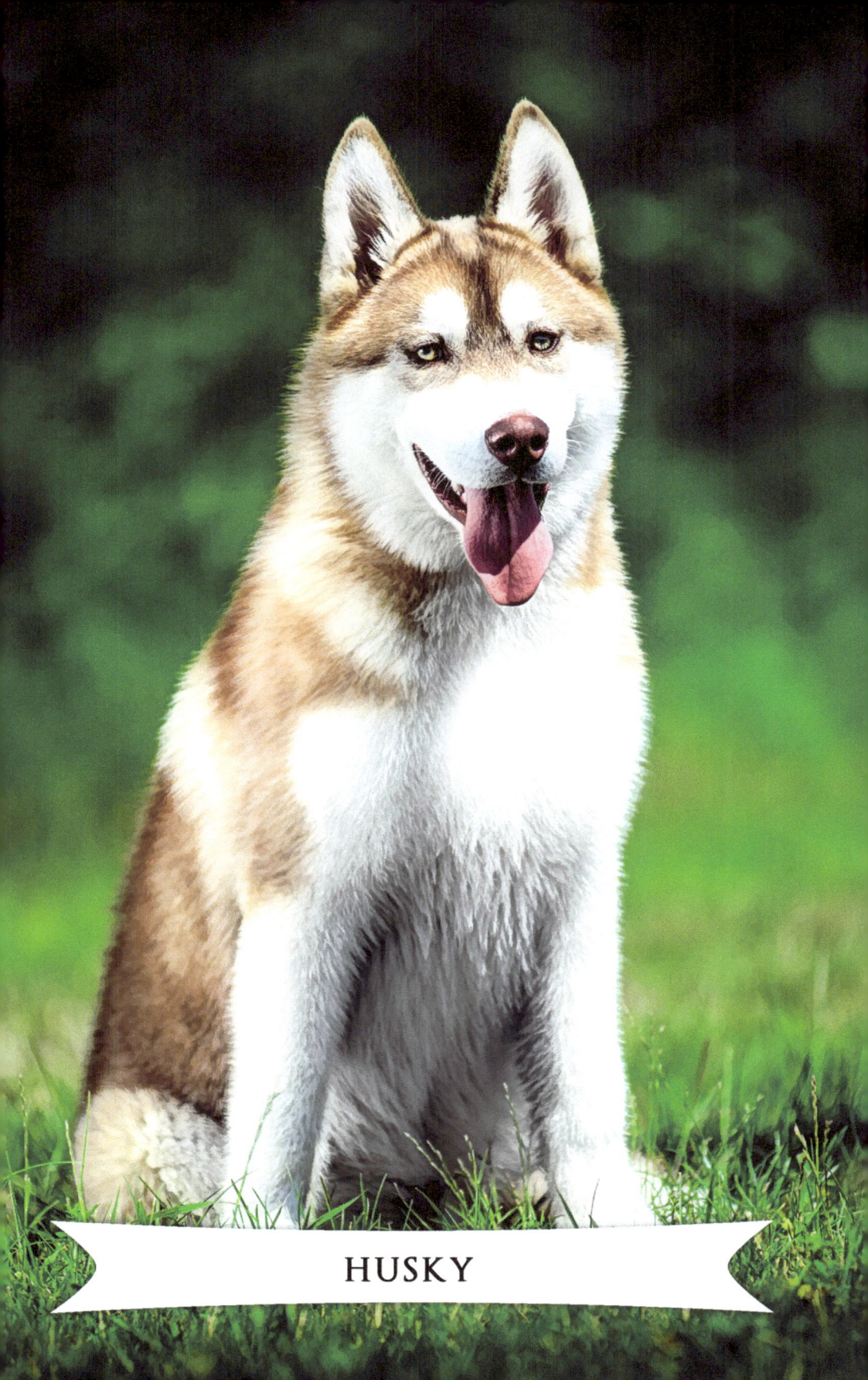

HUSKY

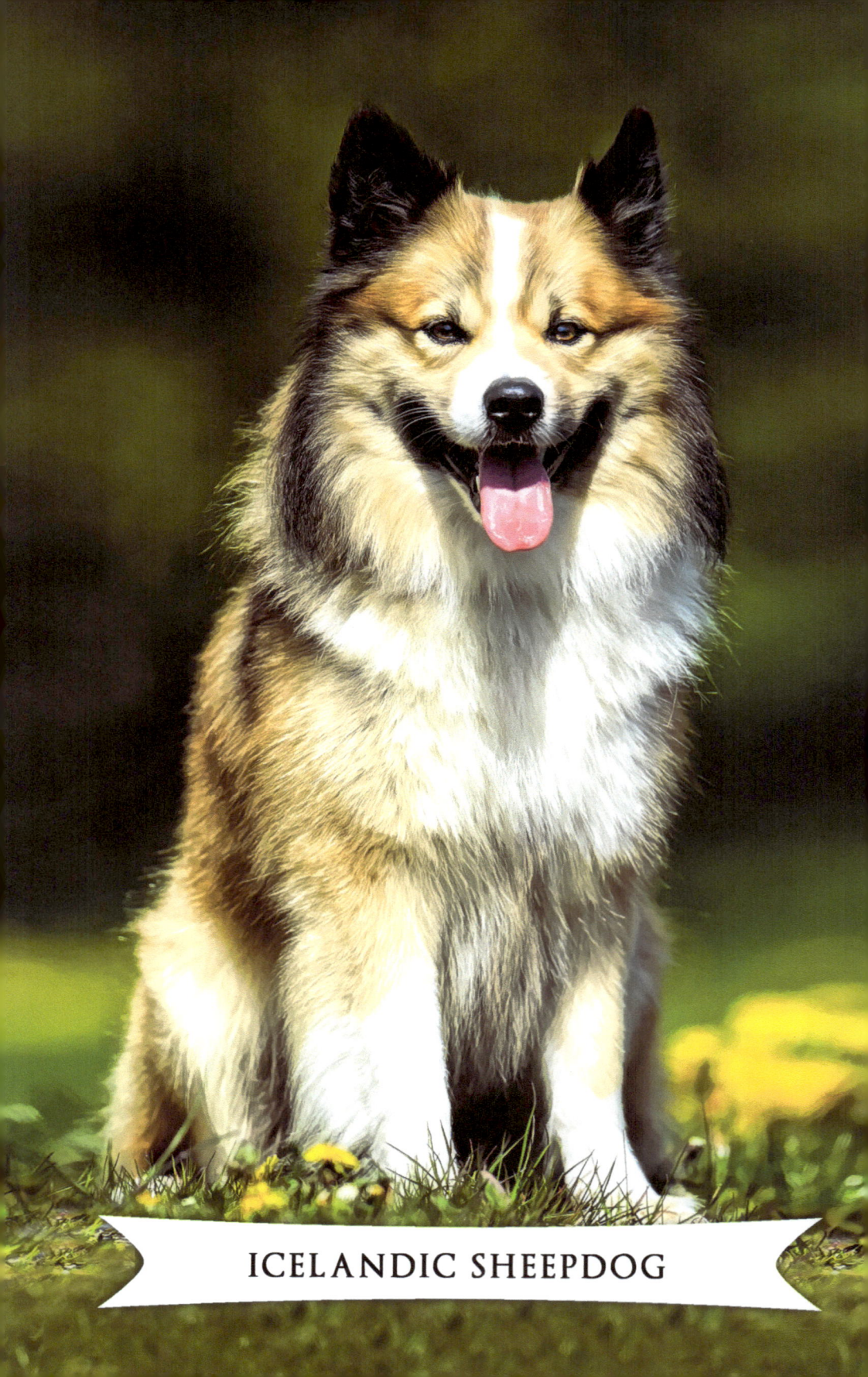

ICELANDIC SHEEPDOG

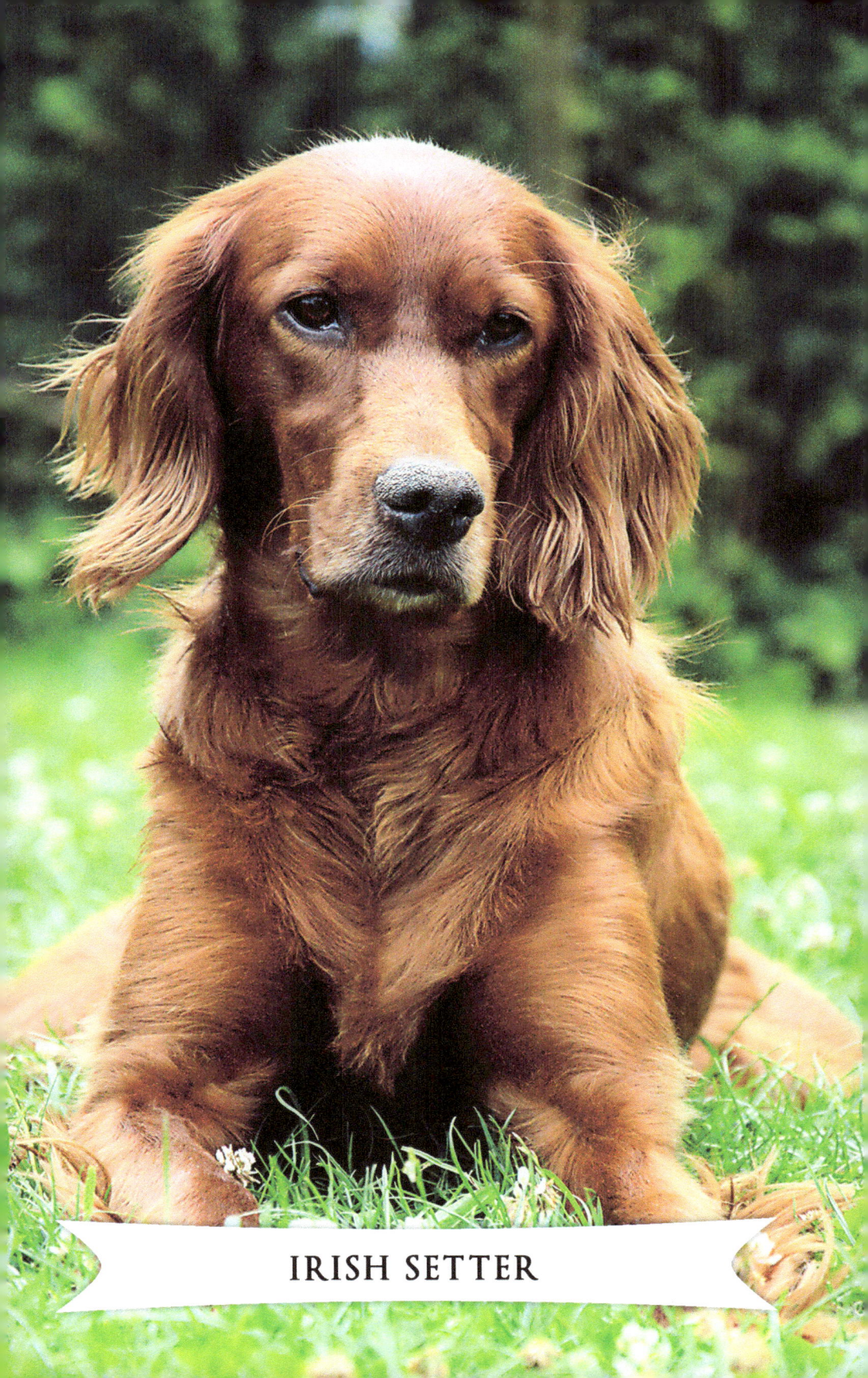

IRISH SETTER

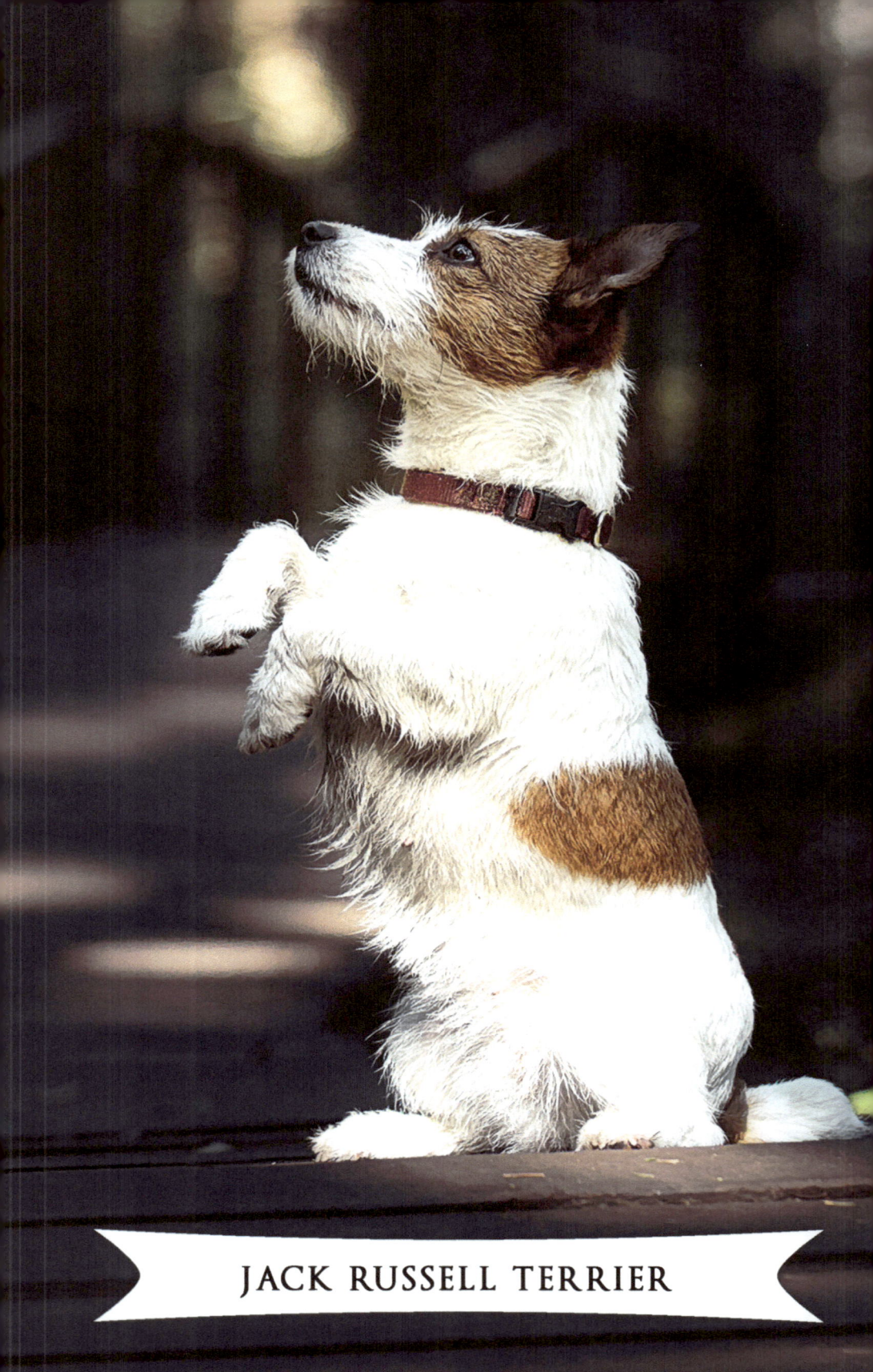

JACK RUSSELL TERRIER

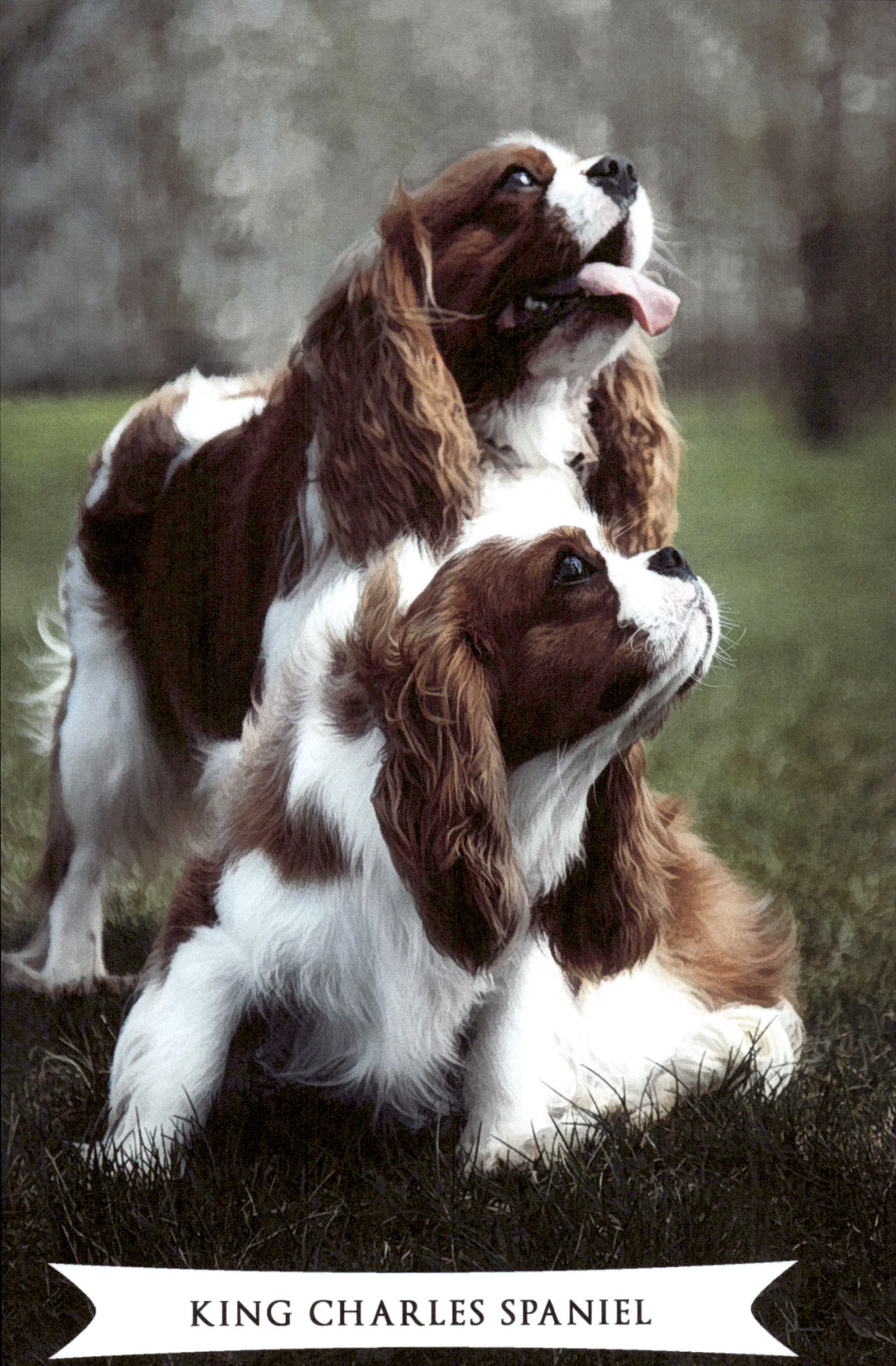

KING CHARLES SPANIEL

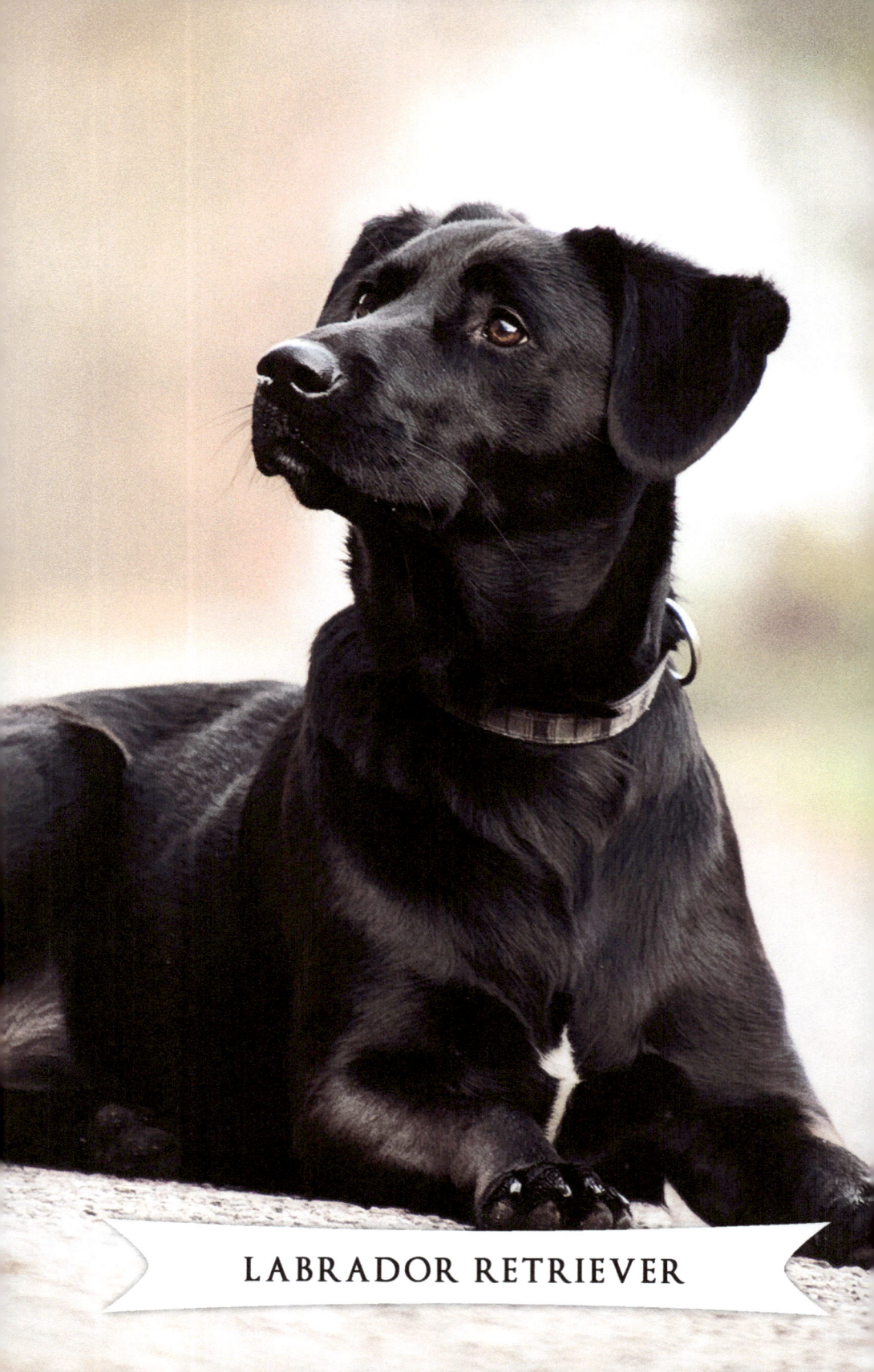

LABRADOR RETRIEVER

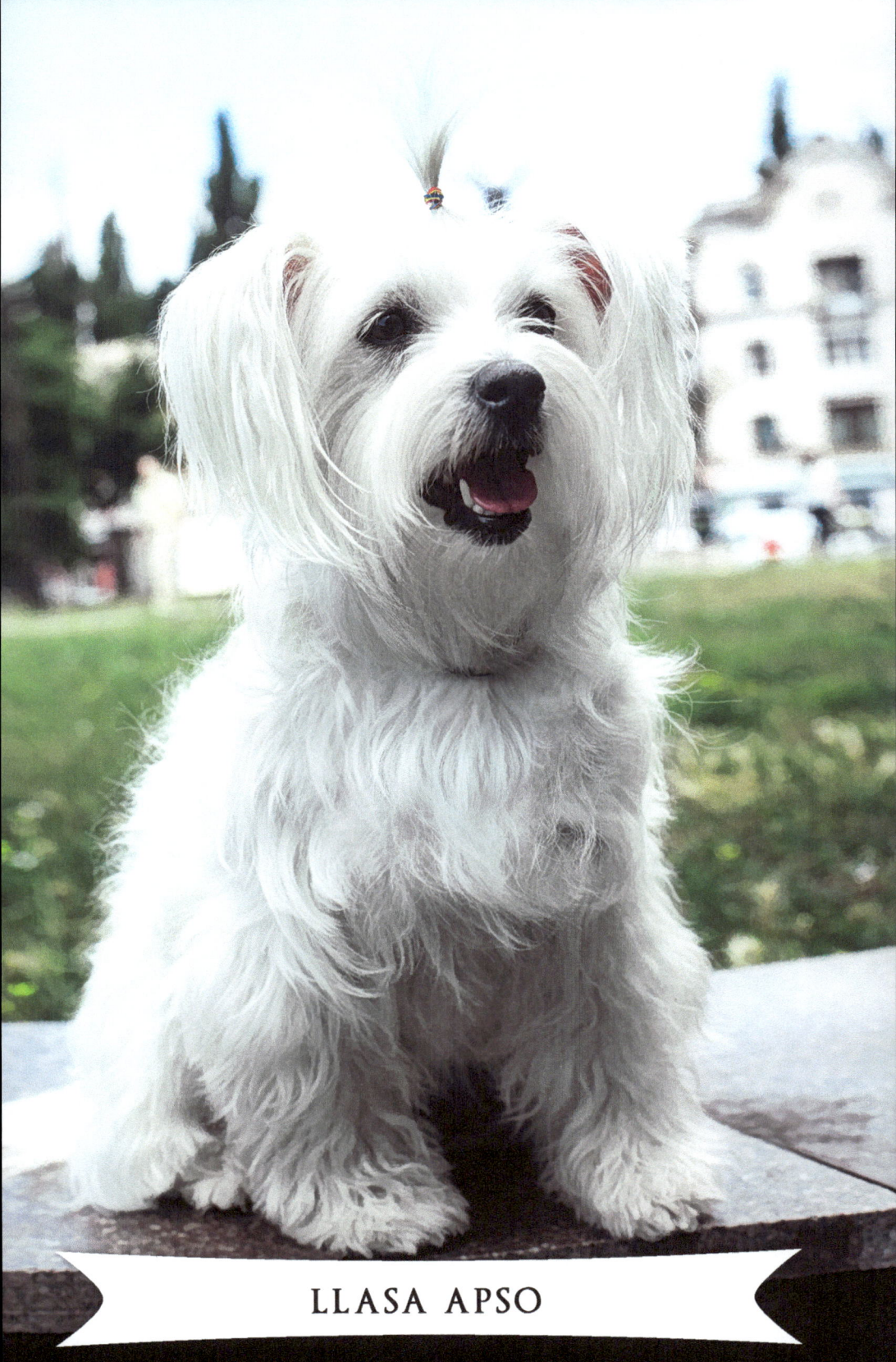

LLASA APSO

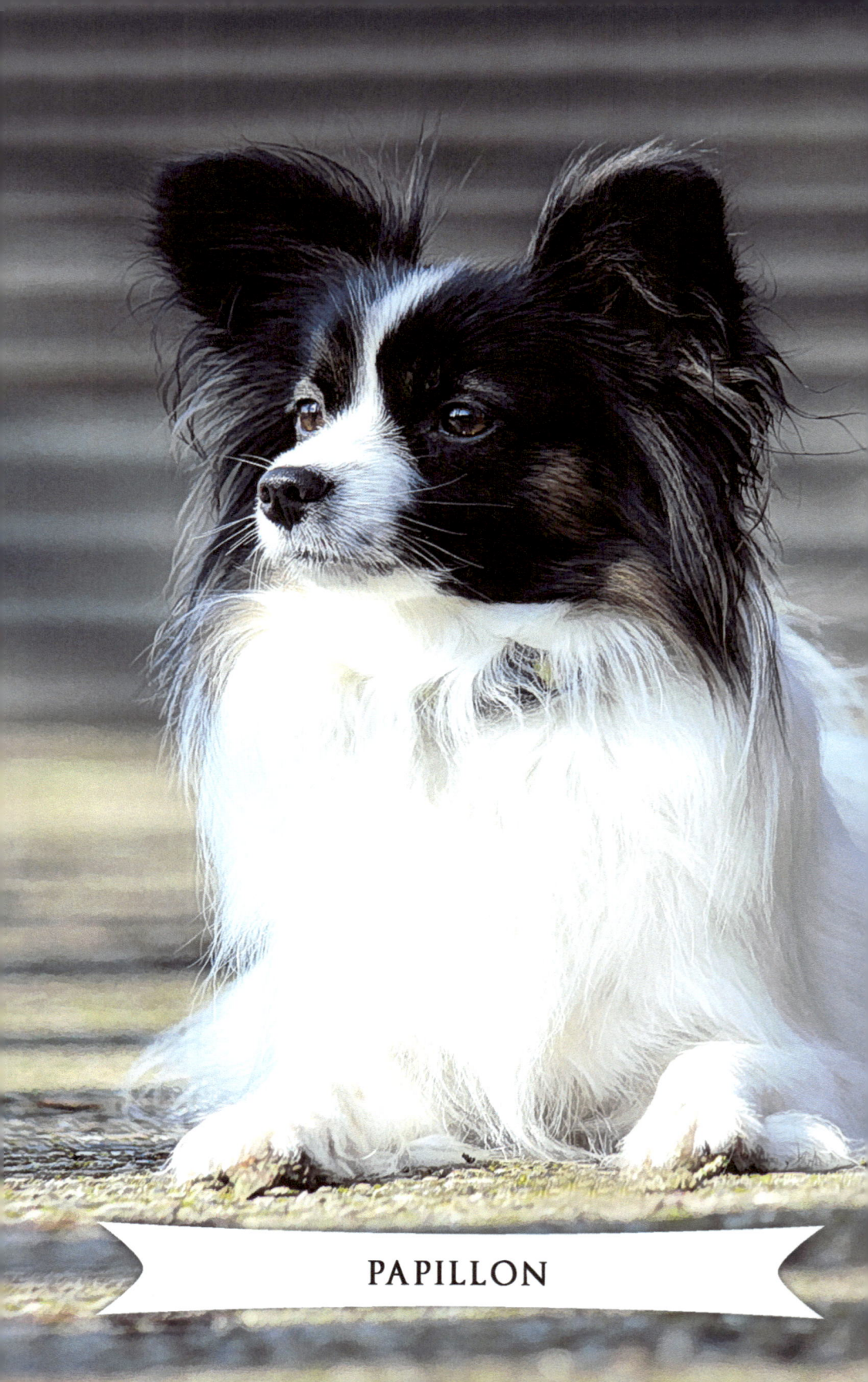

PAPILLON

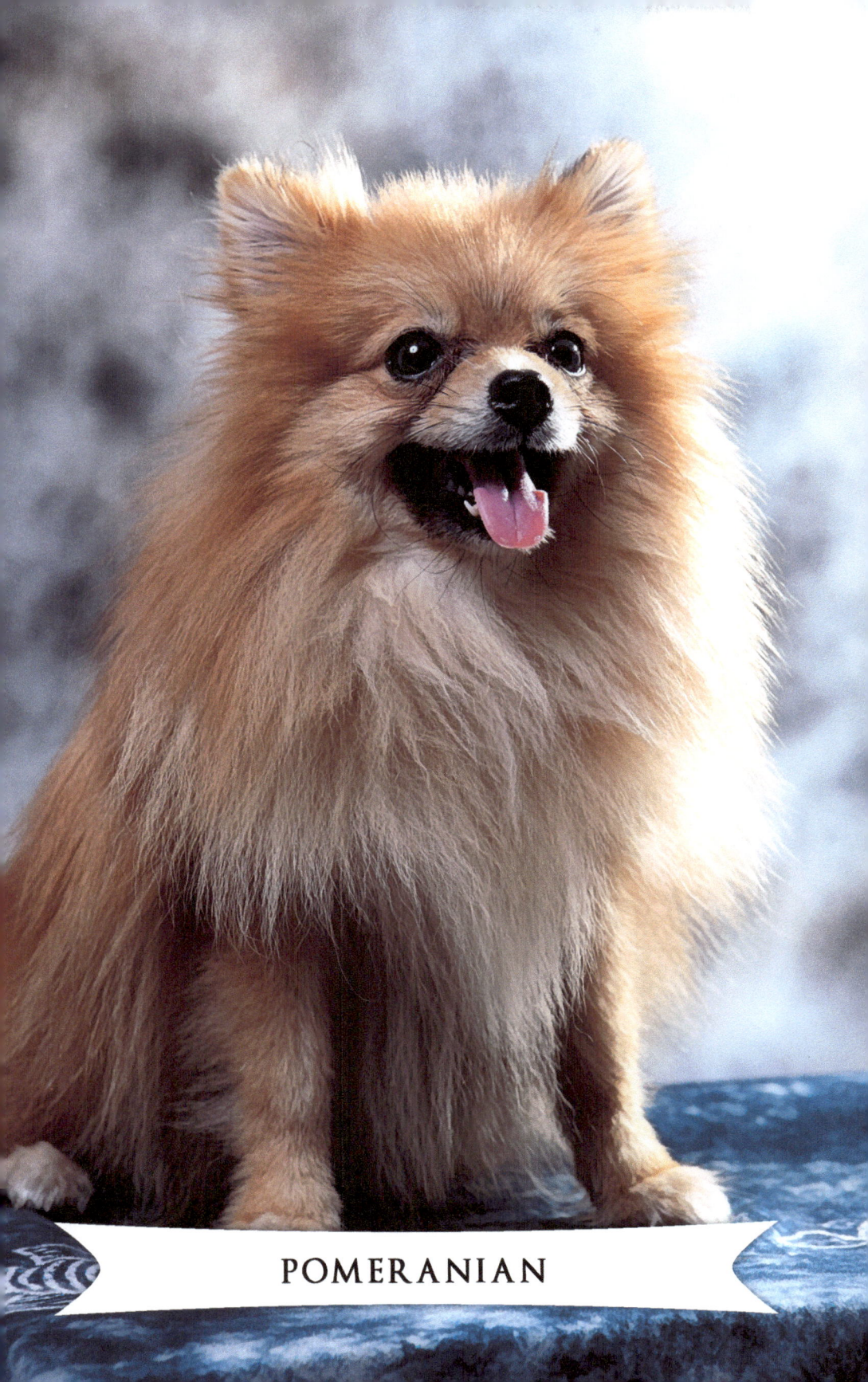

POMERANIAN

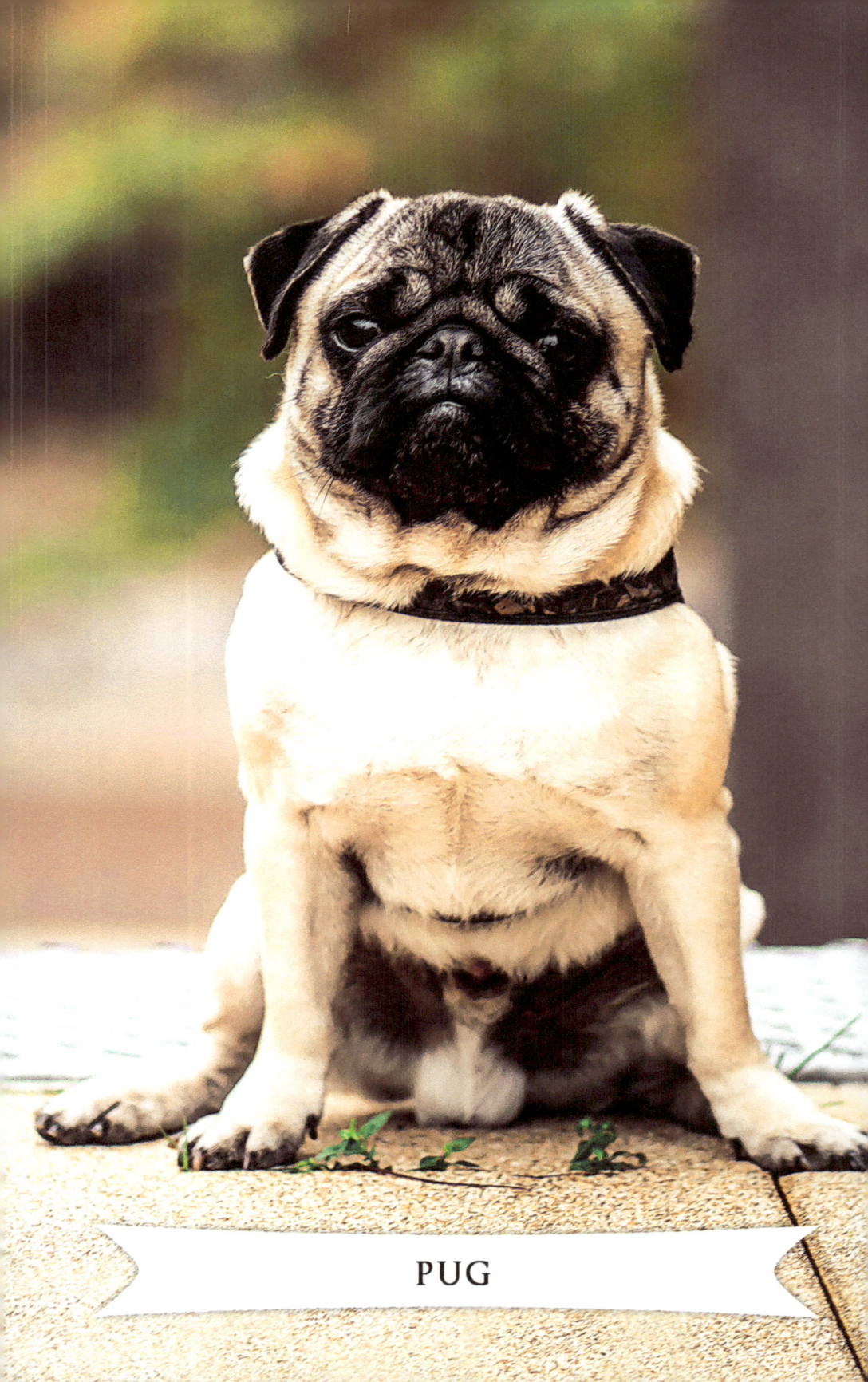

PUG

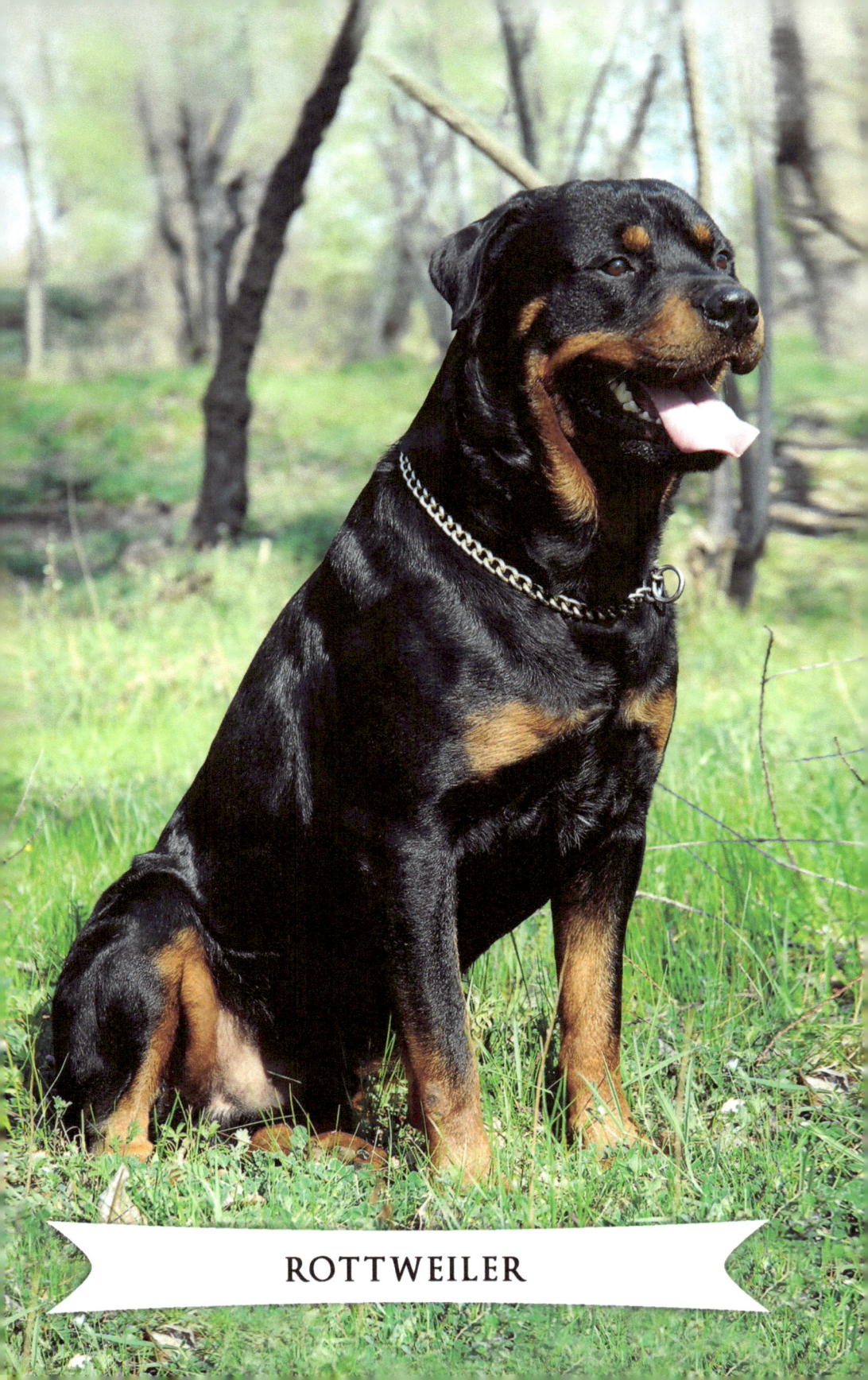

ROTTWEILER

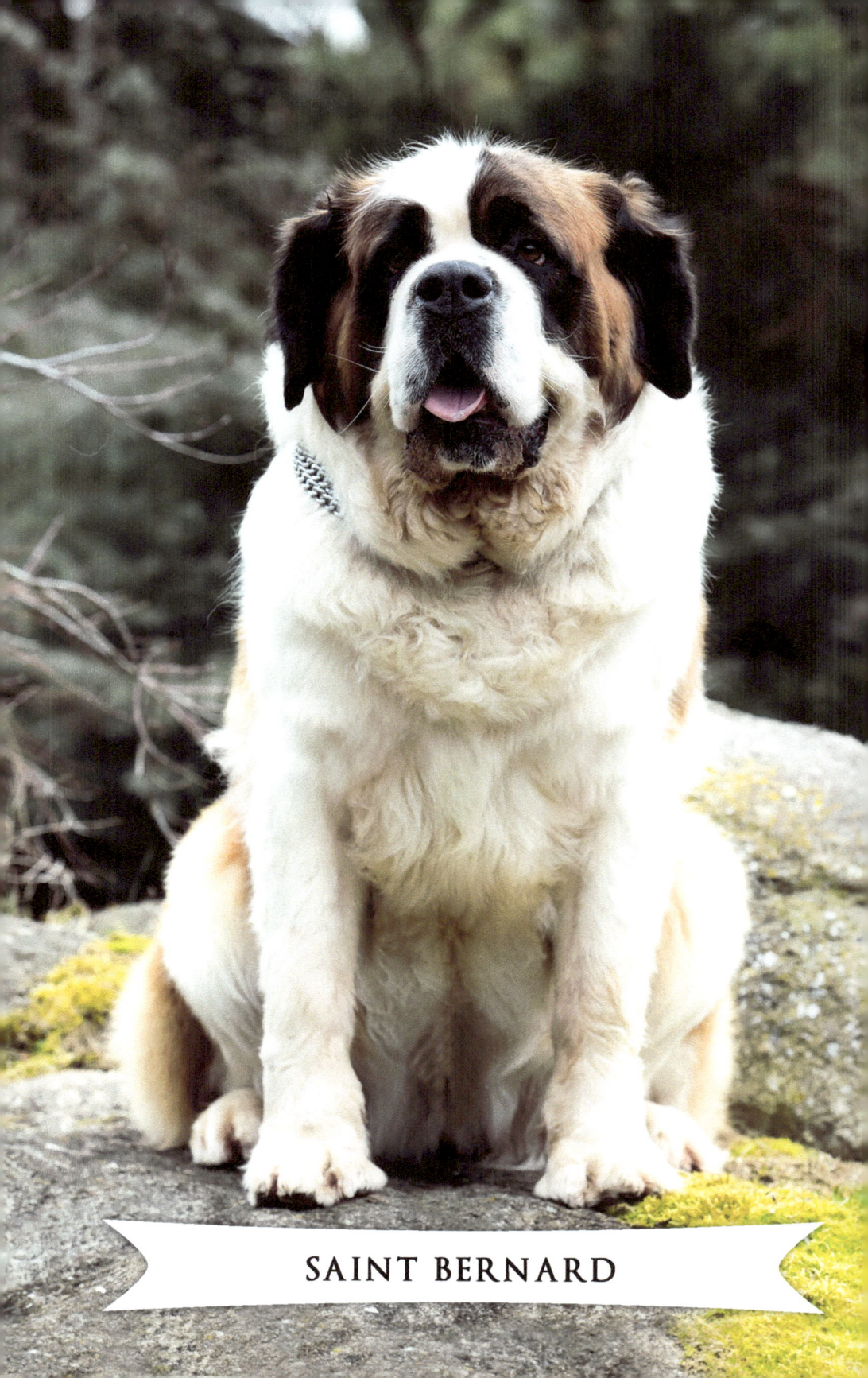

SAINT BERNARD

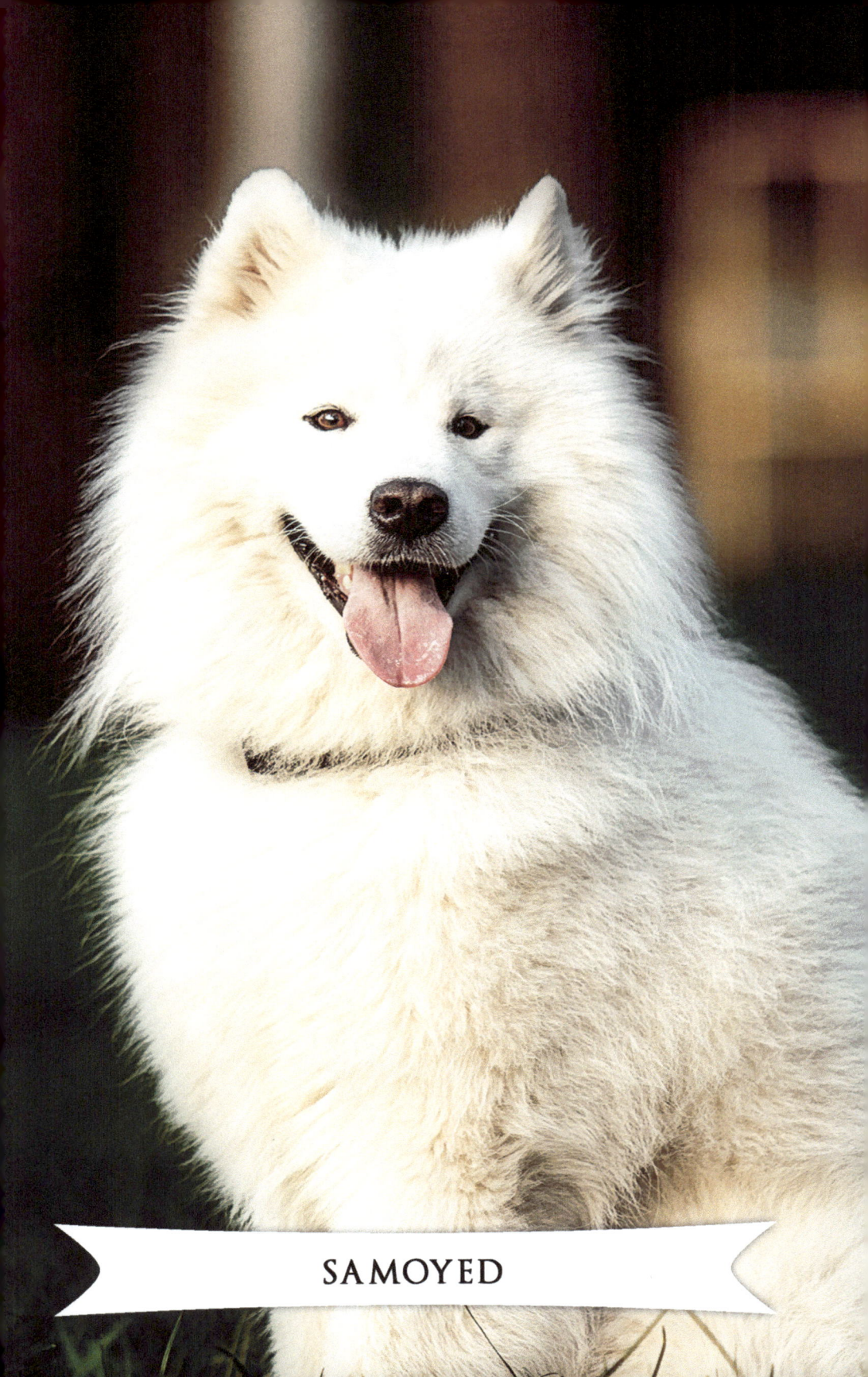

SAMOYED

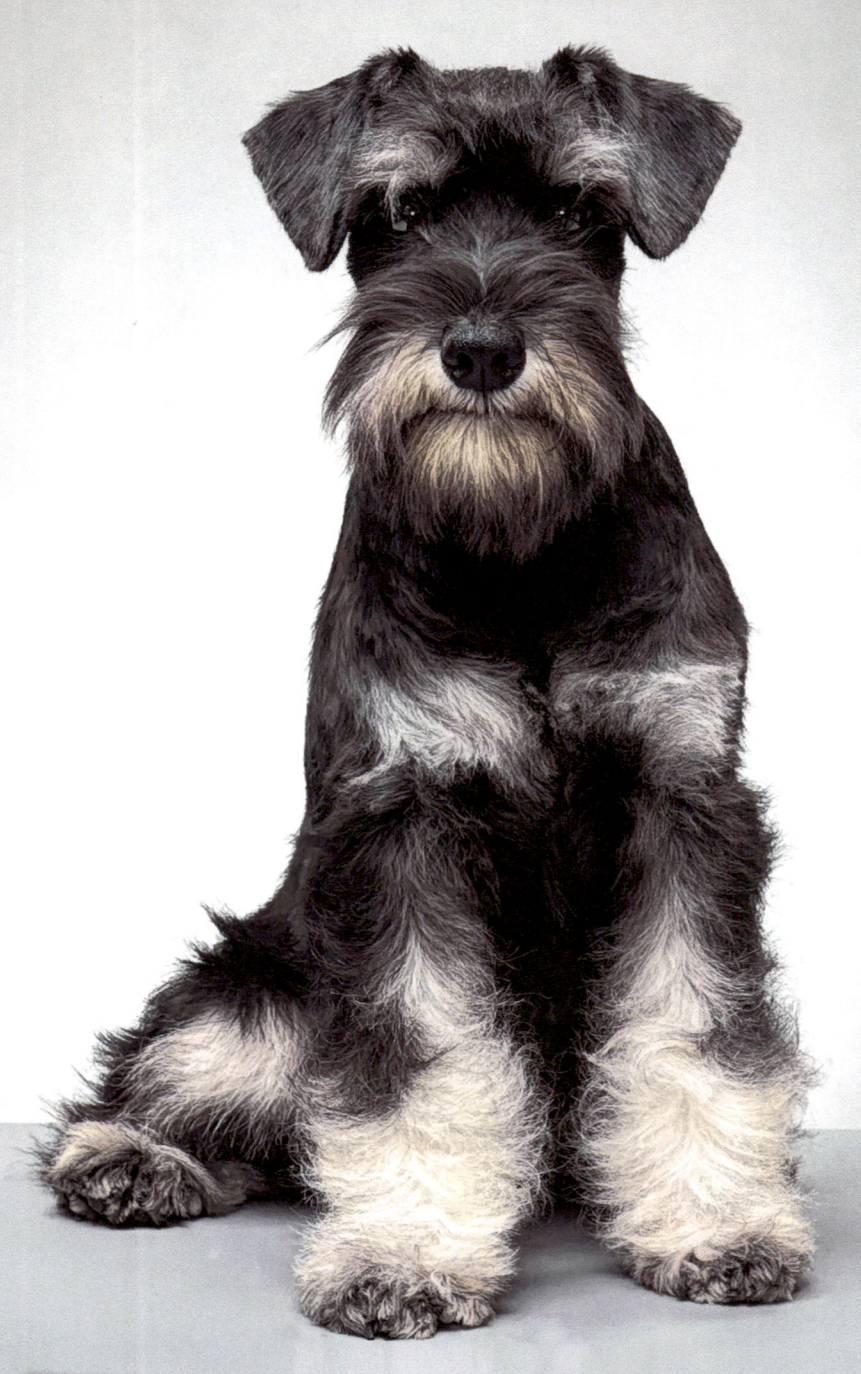

SCHNAUZER

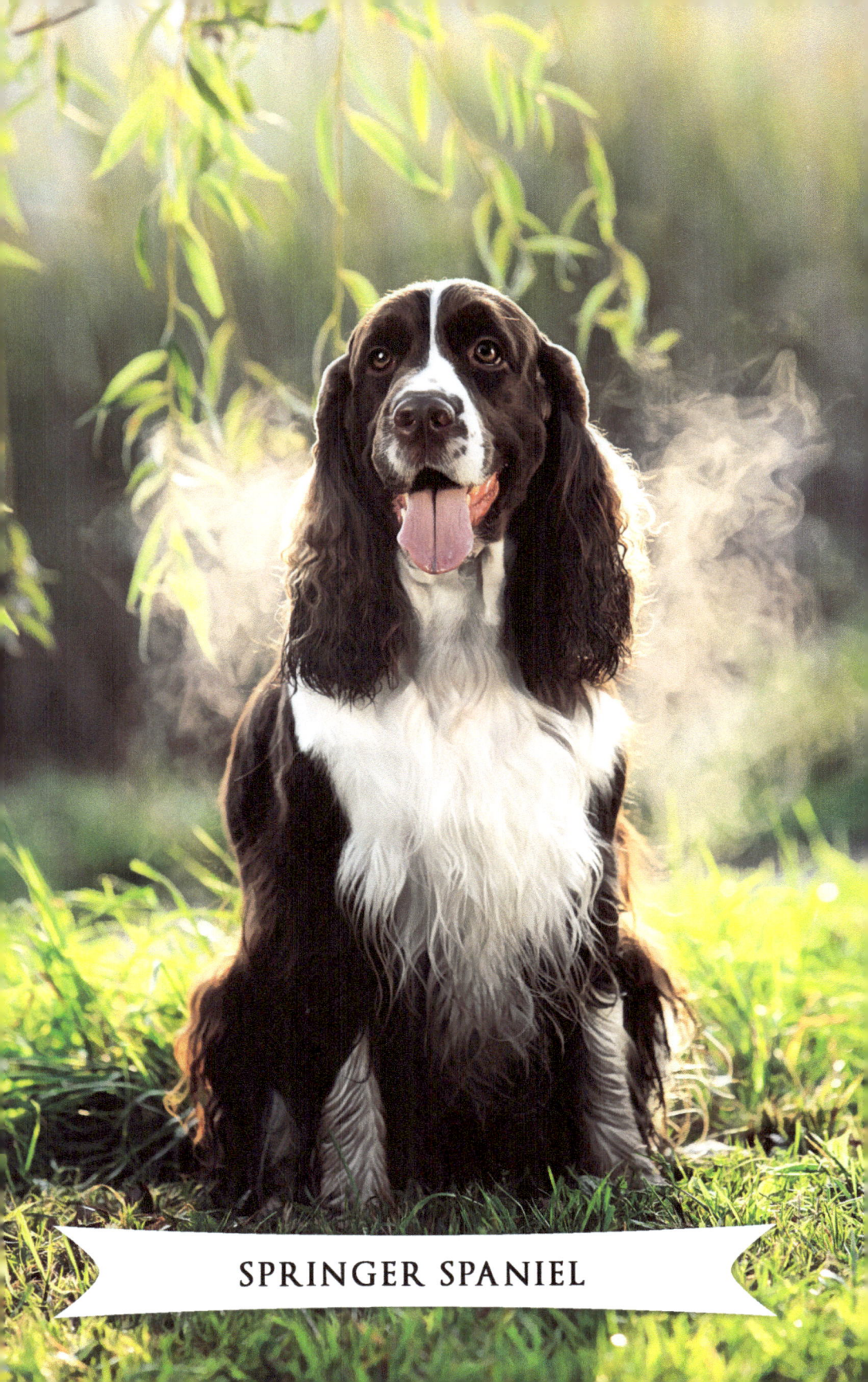

SPRINGER SPANIEL

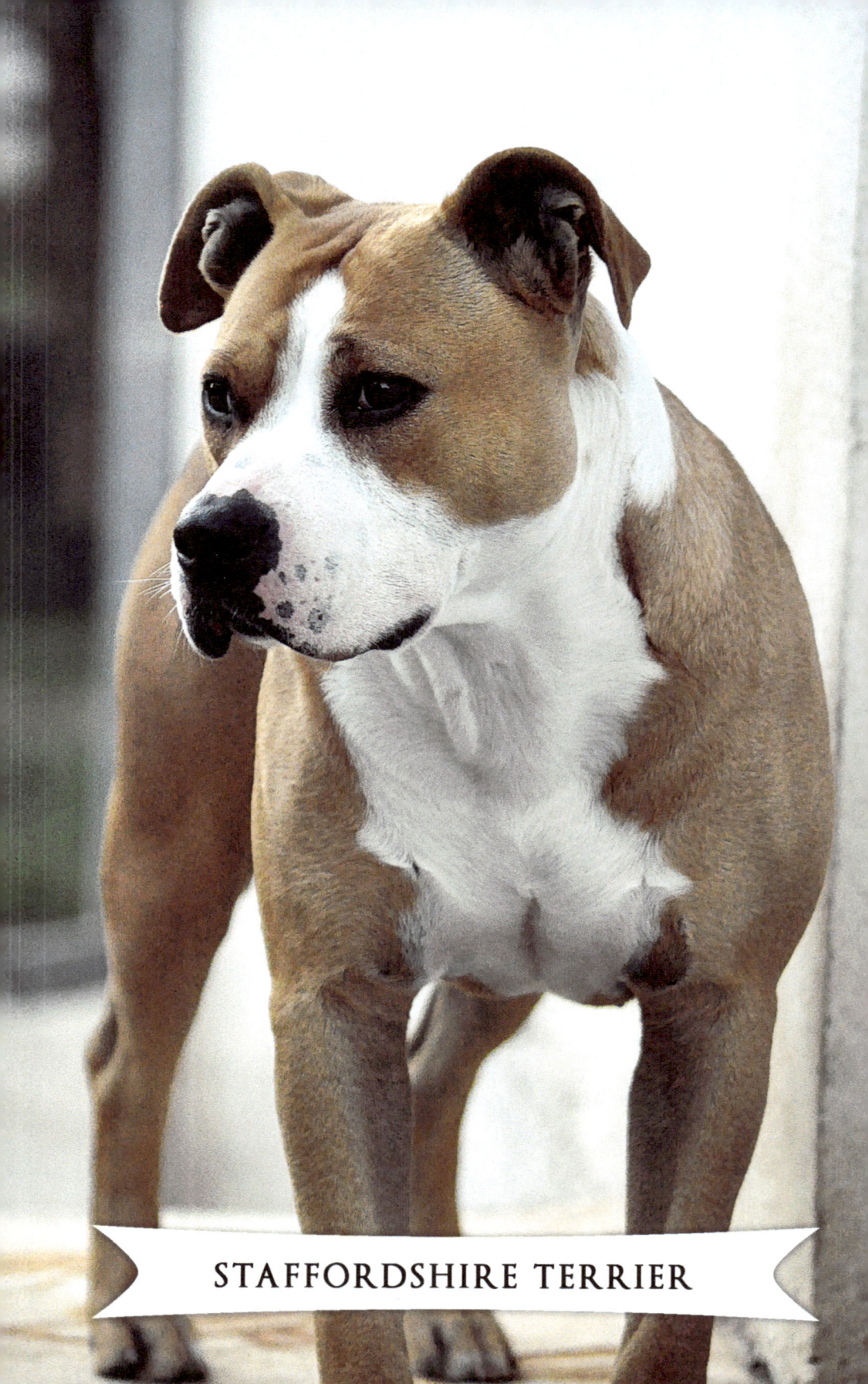

STAFFORDSHIRE TERRIER

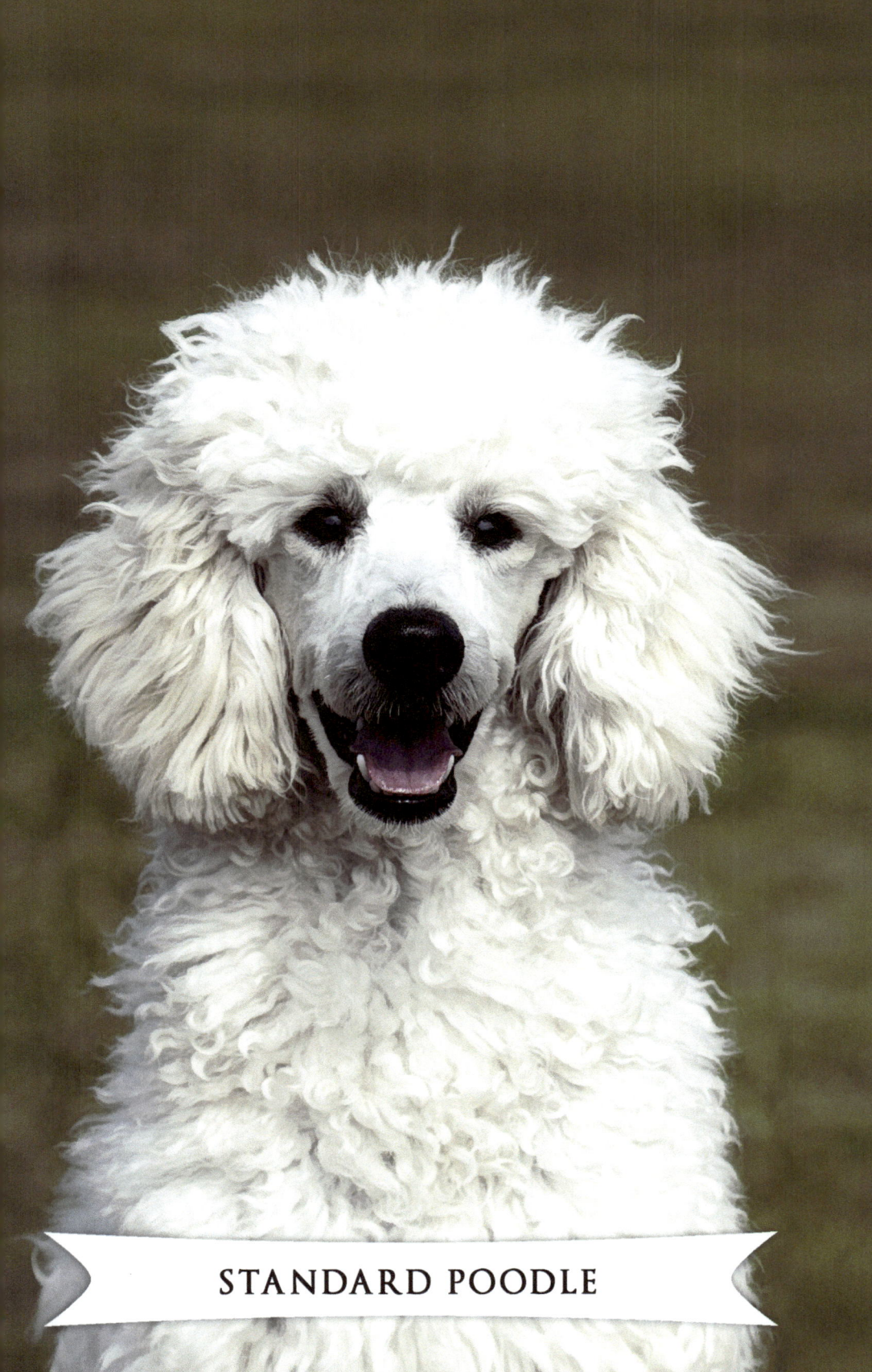

STANDARD POODLE

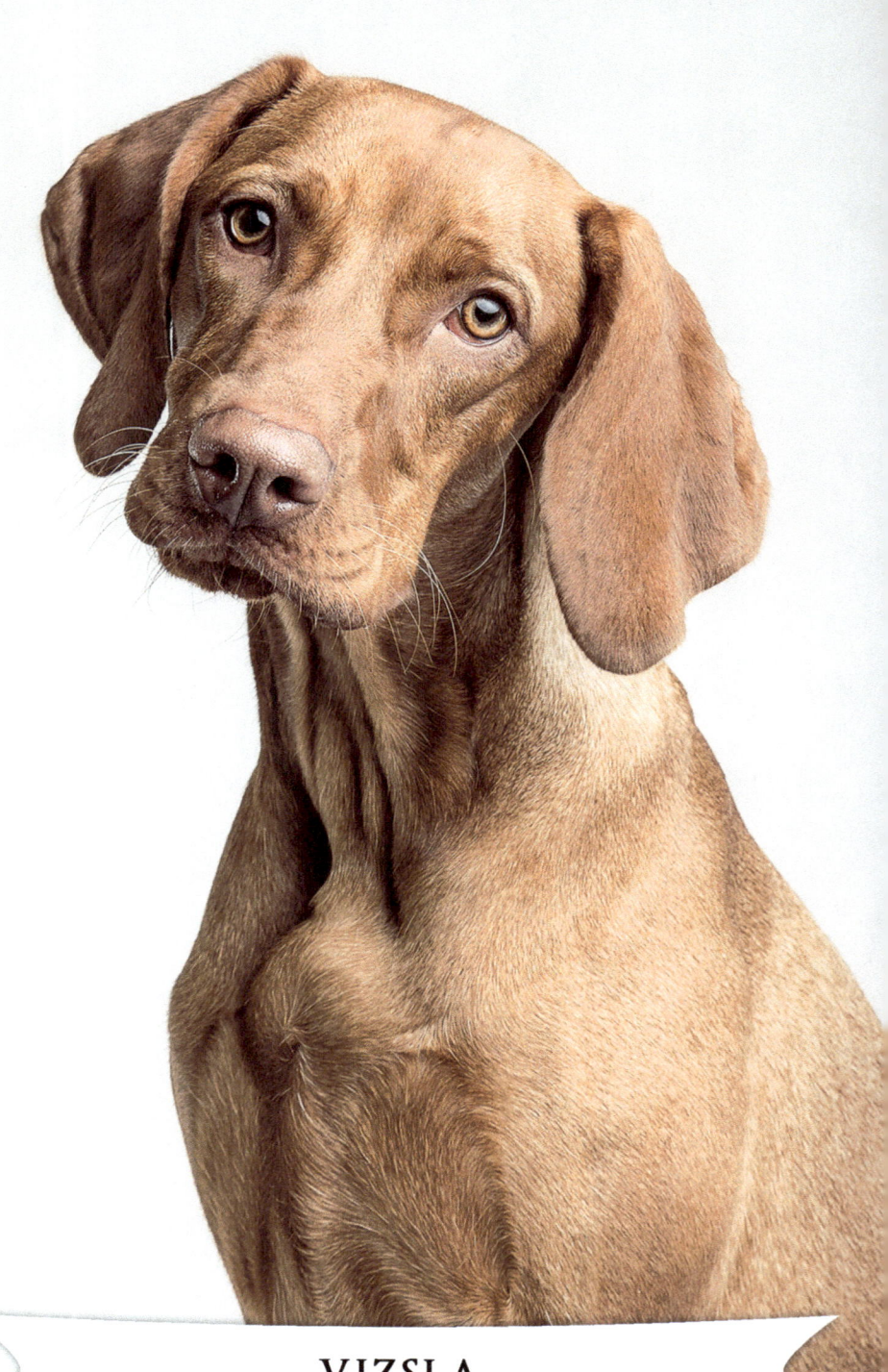

VIZSLA

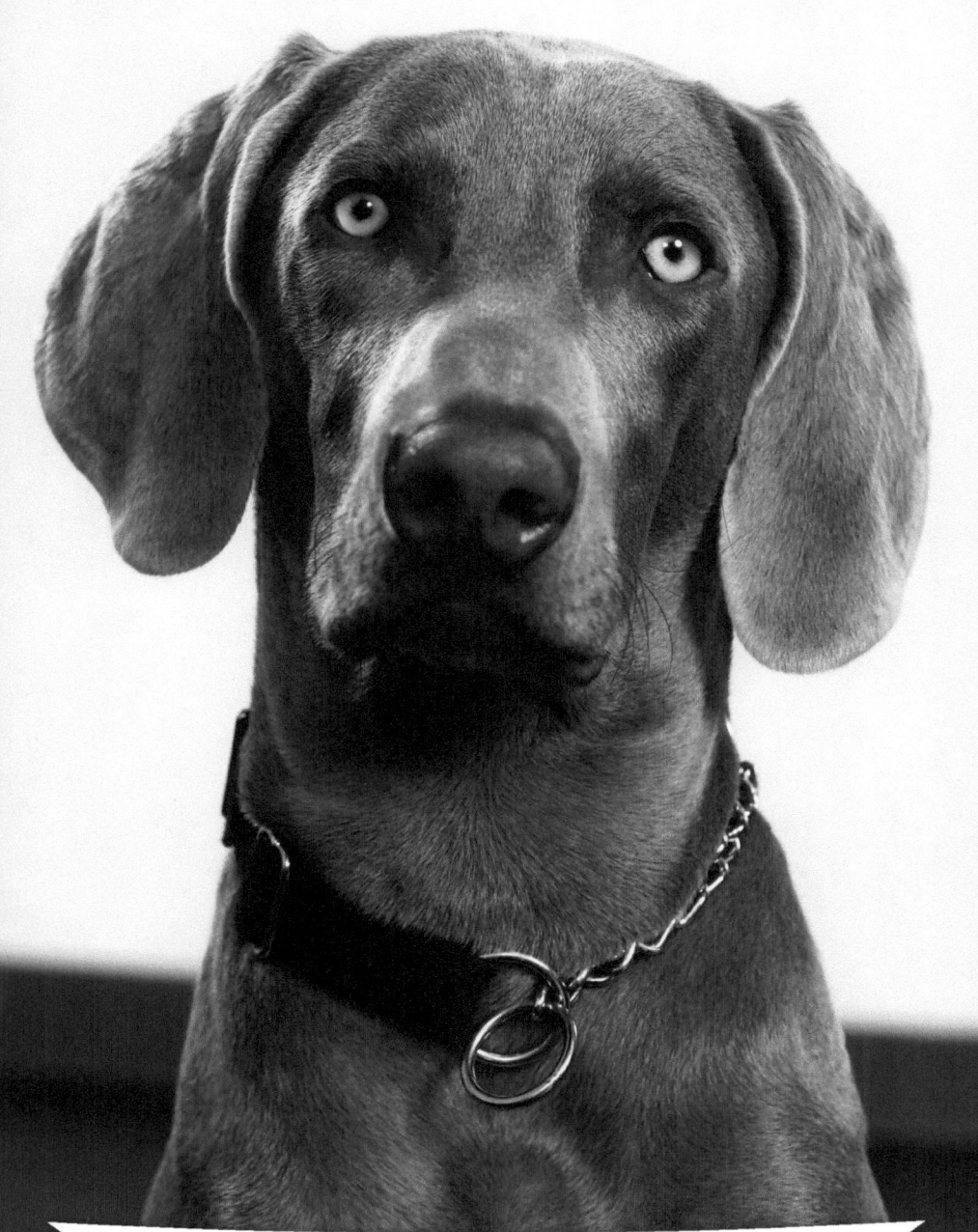

WEIMARANER

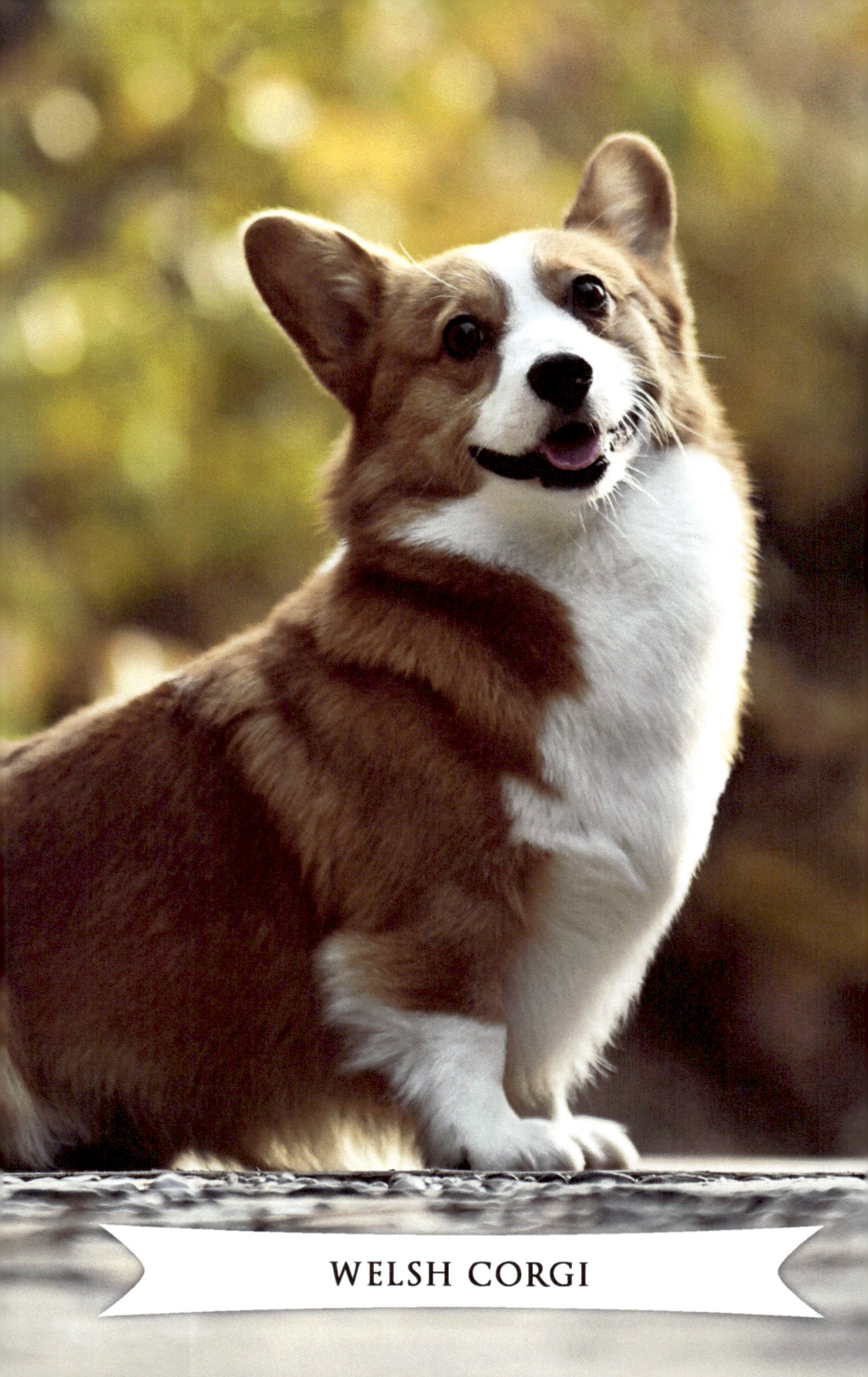

WELSH CORGI

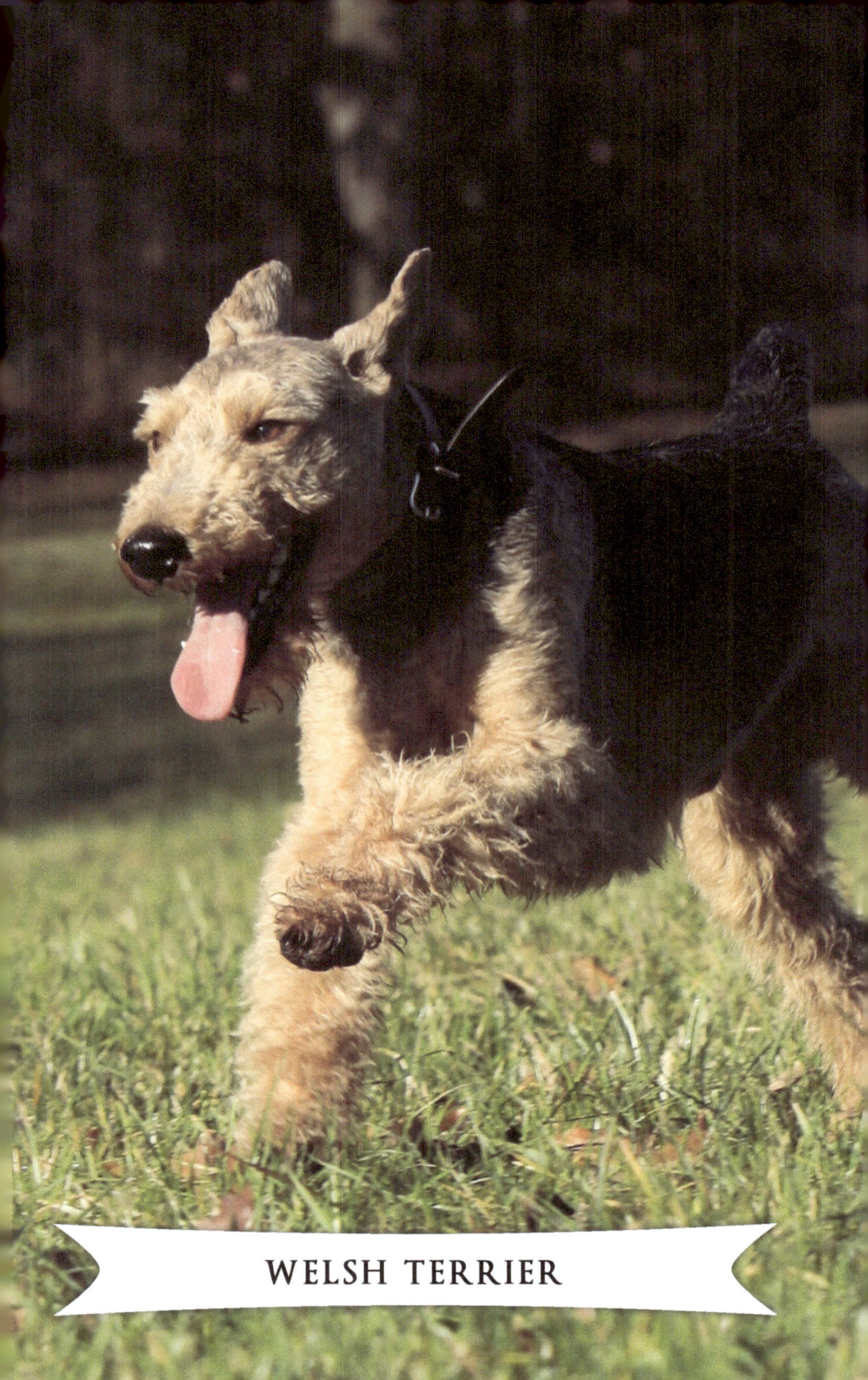

WELSH TERRIER

www.ingramcontent.com/pod-product-compliance
Lightning Source LLC
Chambersburg PA
CBHW050757290526
45792CB00008B/2219